T0344608

Scientific Basis of the Royal College of Radiologists Fellowship (2nd Edition)

Illustrated questions and answers

IPEM–IOP Series in Physics and Engineering in Medicine and Biology

About the Series
Series in Physics and Engineering in Medicine and Biology will allow IPEM to enhance its mission to 'advance physics and engineering applied to medicine and biology for the public good.'

Focusing on key areas including, but not limited to:

- clinical engineering
- diagnostic radiology
- informatics and computing
- magnetic resonance imaging
- nuclear medicine
- physiological measurement
- radiation protection
- radiotherapy
- rehabilitation engineering
- ultrasound and non-ionizing radiation.

A number of IPEM–IOP titles are published as part of the EUTEMPE Network Series for Medical Physics Experts.

Scientific Basis of the Royal College of Radiologists Fellowship (2nd Edition)

Illustrated questions and answers

Malcolm Sperrin
Oxford University Hospitals, Oxford, UK

John Winder
RJ Imaging, Belfast, UK

IOP Publishing, Bristol, UK

ISBN   978-0-7503-2148-8 (ebook)
ISBN   978-0-7503-2146-4 (print)
ISBN   978-0-7503-2149-5 (myPrint)
ISBN   978-0-7503-2147-1 (mobi)

DOI   10.1088/978-0-7503-2148-8

Version: 20191101

IOP ebooks

British Library Cataloguing-in-Publication Data: A catalogue record for this book is available from the British Library.

Published by IOP Publishing, wholly owned by The Institute of Physics, London

IOP Publishing, Temple Circus, Temple Way, Bristol, BS1 6HG, UK

US Office: IOP Publishing, Inc., 190 North Independence Mall West, Suite 601, Philadelphia, PA 19106, USA

Contents

3   Imaging theory   3-1

Introduction

Science and medicine have long been close partners. This is particularly true in radiology where the availability of imaging techniques is central to diagnosis. In its simplest sense, imaging can be thought of as a technique which uses some measurable parameter of the patient to provide a basis for contrast in an image and the science is the connection between the patient and the image.

However, science is far more than just providing a vehicle for understanding an imaging or therapeutic process. An understanding of the science underlying a process enables the right person to develop new techniques, understand imaging limitations and develop a portfolio of research.

A knowledge of scientific principles is also mandated as a result of a need to understand best and safest practice especially in the use of ionizing radiation where legislation, guidance and risk all form part of medical specialists' pressures at work.

It is no surprise therefore that radiologists are obliged to study and pass physics exams. Such exams do present a considerable challenge and the authors of this work recognise and sympathise with that challenge and have set about to create a volume which is intended to be an educational resource and not just a pre-exam 'crammer'. Both authors have considerable experience in teaching, supporting and examining in medical science and have developed an awareness of where those sitting professional exams have traditionally struggled. This text is a distillation of that experience.

The text itself is arranged in a manner to encourage learning and understanding of the key concepts rather than just provide a vehicle to pass the exams. The images and diagrams which accompany each question should provide a stimulus to the concepts being challenged rather than be directed related to the question. The answers also contain some explanation that in many instances goes beyond a simple explanation to support true/false.

The authors hope that the text continues to be used beyond the awarding of Fellowship to the reader and future revisions will include updates, new questions and feedback from those who have found the book to be a usable resource.

Professor Malcolm Sperrin   Dr John Winder
Oxford University Hosptals   RJ Imaging
Oxford   Belfast

Author biographies

Malcolm Sperrin

 Malcolm Sperrin was born in Cuba of diplomatic parents in 1963, and attended The Harvey Grammar School in Folkestone leaving there in 1981 to study Physics with Maths at Reading University. His first job was working on Artificial Intelligence and then with the UK Atomic Energy Authority on reactor fault analysis. This experience placed him in a good position to provide insight into both the Chernobyl and Fukushima incidents.

After further study at Reading University, Malcolm joined Medical Physics at the Churchill Hospital in Oxford with responsibility for non-ionizing radiation. In 1995, Malcolm moved to the Princess Margaret Hospital in Swindon acting as Deputy Head of Department and then, in 2002, he moved to The Royal Berkshire Hospital in Reading taking on the role of Departmental Director. More recently Malcolm moved to the Oxford University Hospitals as Director of Medical Physics and Clinical Engineering and Trust Lead Scientist.

Malcolm has a special interest in radiation medicine, especially Nuclear Medicine and Radiotherapy. He also plays a significant role in radiation protection and contingency planning. In parallel to his conventional hospital duties, Malcolm also spends a lot of time teaching and lecturing with organisations including Oxford Postgraduate Medical School, The Open University and various Royal Colleges not to mention lectureships at Guildford and the University of the West of England.

Malcolm was made visiting Professor at Reading, Guildford and Open Universities and visiting academic at Oxford University and plays a role on the national stage with the Institute of Physics, Royal Institution, Science Media Centre and the British Association for the Advancement of Science. Malcolm also feeds into activities centred on science and health policy at the DoH.

Malcolm's down-to-earth approach to Medical Science has led to him being frequently sought by the media for comment on mobile phone use, WiFi safety and even the risks from the Fukushima reactor. He is very active in developing innovation whether operational or scientific and has recently been involved in initiatives with Microsoft and other multi-national companies with a drive to improve patient outcomes.

Malcolm is a keen adventure sports enthusiast and likes to climb, cave and canoe and has been known to parachute. He has a partner, Nicki (who is not sure about the parachuting), an 9-year-old son and a spaniel called Harvey.

John Winder

 Dr John Winder was born in Belfast, United Kingdom and attended the University of Ulster from 1980 to 1983 studying Physics and Chemistry in a Combined Science degree. He subsequently completed a Master of Science in Physics of the Atmosphere at University College of Wales, Aberystwyth, in 1985 and was awarded a PhD entitled '3D medical imaging and rapid prototyping' in 2004 by the University of Ulster.

After working as a Research Assistant in Physics at Queens University of Belfast, he became a Clinical Scientist (medical physics) at the Royal Victoria Hospital, Belfast. After training he became a Member of the Institute of Physics and Engineering in Medicine in 1992 and gained his Fellowship in 2014. In 1992, John became the first MR physicist for Northern Ireland, as well as providing scientific and research support to Radiology. He was the physics tutor for the Northern Ireland Part 1 Radiology Training Fellowship and taught on the programme for 15 years. He was a member of the Royal College of Radiologists Physics Working Group from 2008 to 2012 and was awarded honorary membership of the College in 2013.

John worked at The University of Ulster from 2002 until 2017 as a Reader in Healthcare Science as a lecturer and researcher, contributing to the Healthcare Science and Radiography programmes. His research interests are in 3D medical imaging, rapid prototyping (3D printing) and has published over 100 research papers, 7 book chapters and supervised 11 PhD students. He is known for his clear communication of science and has been guest speaker at a range of UK Radiology and other clinical conferences.

John is self-employed at RJ imaging, Belfast, and works on scientific writing and creating customised anatomical models for the Northern Ireland National Health Service.

IOP Publishing

Scientific Basis of the Royal College of Radiologists Fellowship (2nd Edition)

Illustrated questions and answers

Malcolm Sperrin and John Winder

Chapter 1

Basic physics

Imaging is a physical process in which aspects of the patients' tissues are used to generate different signals which in turn provide contrast in a final image. The nature of the contrast is derived from how the tissue interacts with the radiation used and hence a knowledge of energy levels, atomic structures along with many other concepts is essential in order to understand both the general concepts and finer subtleties

doi:10.1088/978-0-7503-2148-8ch1

1-1

of how the imaging process takes place. In addition to image formation, safety and image optimisation can only be properly understood if the underlying physical processes are clear. The level at which it is necessary to understand the physics is not great for the part 1 Fellowship. There is no expectation of being able to remember complex equations or extensive derivations; rather, it is sufficient to be conversant with the scientific principles at GCSE or early stage 'A' level. There are many texts available as well as help on the internet if you need any refreshing on such concepts.

Q1.1 The structure of the atom

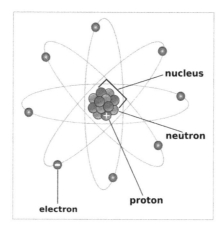

The accepted and simple structure of the atom shows it consists of two parts, a nucleus made of nucleons (protons and neutrons) and a circling cloud of negatively charged particles called electrons. This was established by the physicist Neils Bohr in 1913. The nucleus is bound very tightly together by a force known as the nuclear force, whilst electrons are held in orbit by the electromagnetic (EM) force.

The vast majority of the mass of atoms lies within the nucleus (electron mass is 1/1840 of one nucleon). The mass number (A) defines the number of nucleons for a particular element, whilst the atomic number (Z) defines the number of protons or electrons. Electrons exist at clearly defined energy levels around the nucleus called electron shells. Ionization is the process where an atom or molecule becomes charged due to a change in its structure, such as the loss of some electrons. Ionized particles are highly chemically reactive and therefore may cause problems within the body's biochemistry.

Concerning the structure of the atom (true or false)
    a. Carbon has a mass number of 12 and an atomic number of 6, it has 6 neutrons.
    b. The most common form of oxygen has an atomic number of 16.
    c. Ionization is defined as the loss of some neutrons from the nucleus.
    d. High energy x-rays bombarding an atom cause ionization by knocking out shell electrons on the target material.
    e. Electrons are repelled by a negatively charged electric plate.

Answers

a. Carbon has a mass number of 12 and an atomic number of 6, it has 6 neutrons.

   True: The carbon nucleus comprises 6 neutrons and 6 protons, giving rise to a total of 12 nucleons. There are exceptions such as isotopes where, for a given element, the number of neutrons will differ but the number of protons will stay the same, giving rise to a range of atomic masses for a given element, for example carbon-13 has 6 protons but 7 neutrons. Other characteristics such as nuclear magnetic moment will also vary between isotopes.

b. The most common form of oxygen has an atomic number of 16.

   False: Oxygen has an atomic mass of 16 (the atomic number is 8).

c. Ionization is defined as the loss of some neutrons from the nucleus.

   False: Ionization is a process by which neutral atoms or molecules gain or lose electrons acquiring a net charge. Ionization may be caused by heat, radiation, chemical reactions or electrical discharge.

d. High energy x-rays bombarding an atom cause ionization by knocking out shell electrons on the target material.

   True: Incident photons can have sufficient energy to remove bound electrons leaving the atom with a deficit of electrons and hence it becomes ionized.

e. Electrons are repelled by a negatively charged electric plate.

   True: Electrons have a negative charge and therefore will be repelled by negatively charged plates, for example within an x-ray tube.

Q1.2 Characteristic radiation and atomic shells

Quantum theory explains why electrons can only occupy certain locations within an atom. For instance the innermost shell can only be occupied by two electrons whereas shells further out can contain more electrons. Each of these shells has a well-defined energy and hence any electron transiting from one shell to another is associated with either an absorption or release of energy. This means that for a vacant location in the orbits, an electron dropping into it will release energy in the form of radiation which may be light or x-rays as in the case of characteristic radiation.

Concerning characteristic radiation (true or false)
   a. Electrons require energy to be ejected from an orbital.
   b. All elements have the same K shell energy.
   c. Only wave energy can be used to cause ionization of characteristic energy.
   d. Bremsstrahlung is a manifestation of shell transitions.
   e. Filters utilize shell absorption to optimize radiation dose reduction.

Answers
   a. Electrons require energy to be ejected from an orbital.

   True: As electrons are bound to the nucleus by a force, additional energy must be imparted to the electron that exceeds its binding energy before it is ejected. If insufficient energy is given, the electron may change energy level assuming the deposited energy is sufficient. Otherwise the energy may simply be re-emitted or contribute to heating.

   b. All elements have the same K shell energy.

   False: Each atom has its own energy level which arises from the size and composition of the nucleus. This means that the characteristic radiation is material dependent.

   c. Only x-ray energy can be used to cause ionization leading to photons of characteristic energy.

   False: Heat or particles can also give rise to ionization.

   d. Bremsstrahlung is a manifestation of shell transitions.

   False: Bremsstrahlung arises from the rapid loss of kinetic energy of a charged particle, such as the electrons in an x-ray tube as they hit the anode.

   e. Filters utilize shell absorption to optimize radiation dose reduction.

   True: The presence of the absorption edge means that some energies are preferentially absorbed, hence x-ray photons away from absorption edges will be more heavily absorbed leading to a greater proportion of mono-energetic x-rays in the x-ray spectrum.

Q1.3 The electromagnetic spectrum I

EM radiation can travel through a vacuum and has a constant velocity (3×10^8 m s^{-1}). Note that x-rays and gamma rays have basically the same properties, however, they differ in the source of emission (x-rays from an x-ray tube and gamma rays from radioactive nuclei). They are time varying waves with an electric component and magnetic component which are at right angles to each other. There are different names for EM radiation depending on their individual energies which can be measured in electron volts. Photon energy is proportional to the frequency of the wave and therefore inversely proportional to the wavelength. Radiation with a shorter wavelength, and therefore a higher frequency, has higher photon energy.

Concerning the EM spectrum (true or false)
   a. Infrared (IR) photons have higher energy than ultraviolet (UV) photons.
   b. Molecules vibrate and oscillate in the IR and radio frequency (RF) ranges.
   c. Green light has lower energy photons that blue light.
   d. IR radiation is visible because of its blue hue.
   e. RF radiation is non-ionizing.

Answers
  a. IR photons have higher energy than UV photons.
     False: The energy of EM photons is determined by their frequency. Energy $= h \times f$, where h is Planck's constant and f is frequency. From the figure we can see that IR has a longer wavelength than UV radiation and therefore a lower frequency.
  b. Molecules vibrate and oscillate in the IR and RF ranges.
     True: This occurs because the frequency of the IR/RF photon matches the natural frequency of vibration of the bond between the atoms forming the molecule.
  c. Green light has lower energy photons that blue light.
     True: Using the energy equation above and the wavelengths from the figure, it is clear that blue photons have a shorter wavelength than green photons, therefore a higher frequency and therefore higher energy.
  d. IR radiation is visible because of its blue hue.
     False: The term infra means below (therefore 'below red') and is not visible to the human eye.
  e. RF radiation is non-ionizing.
     True: Although RF radiation photons are not energetic enough to cause ionization, they can cause heating.

Q1.4 The electromagnetic spectrum II

	Non-ionising radiation			Ionising radiation
Type of radiation	extremely low frequency	radio microwave	infrared visible	ultraviolet X-ray Gamma ray
Effects	non-thermal effects?	thermal heating	optical photochemical	broken chemical bonds DNA damage
Source	static or low frequency electric field	radio, tv computer / microwave oven or transmitter	heat lamp, sun, light sources	sun, tannng booths / medical, natural, power station

The EM spectrum extends over many orders of magnitude of frequencies and hence energies. How this energy interacts with matter provides an explanation of how image contrast and radiation risk are calculated and managed.

The ability of a material to attenuate EM radiation is a function of the material's energy levels and how these relate to the energy of the EM radiation. Hence for a given photon, the attenuation will differ between materials, giving rise to a variation in contrast in the final image. This concept also explains the behaviour of the detector where the absorbance in a material gives rise to ionization or heating, both of which can be used to reveal EM interactions.

Concerning the EM spectrum (true or false)
   a. There is an EM energy below which no ionization will occur.
   b. Scatter can occur even if no ionization is present.
   c. UV light does not form part of the EM spectrum.
   d. Gamma rays are particulate in nature because they arise from the particles that constitute the atomic nucleus.
   e. Materials that attenuate at a given energy will always attenuate at lower energies.

Answers

a. There is an EM energy below which no ionization will occur.

True: To cause ionization, the electron must be given sufficient energy to escape from the orbit in which it sits. The orbits have a set amount of energy and this must be exceeded for the electron to escape; this is known as the ionization energy. This energy is different for each element.

b. Scatter can occur even if no ionization is present.

True: An incoming photon may have insufficient energy to ionize an atom but it may change direction or increase the energy of the atom. The photon may then be released as the atom's excess energy is lost resulting in scatter. The atom is excited but not ionized.

c. UV light does not form part of the EM spectrum.

False: UV is an EM phenomenon and the photons carry more energy than visible light since the wavelength is shorter and hence the frequency is higher. However, the energy is usually not sufficient to cause ionization although very high energy UV radiation can cause excitation.

d. Gamma rays are particulate in nature because they arise from the particles that constitute the atomic nucleus.

False: Although the nucleus is particulate in nature, it is the energy levels that are relevant here. As the nucleons relax through one of a number of possible mechanisms, energy can be released in the form of gamma rays.

e. Materials that attenuate at a given energy will always attenuate at lower energies.

False: The photon may have the right energy to be absorbed by the electrons in their orbits leading to ionization or excitation, however, if the photon energy is reduced, they will not have sufficient energy to produce a transition in the atom and hence will not be absorbed. They may undergo scatter.

Q1.5 Luminescence

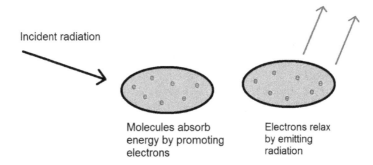

Luminescence is the emission of light from a material that does not derive its energy required for emission from the temperature of the material. For example, phosphorescence, fluorescence and bioluminescence are all forms of luminescence.

A fluorescent material is one that glows or emits light when exposed to radiation, whilst a phosphorescent material is one that keeps glowing after the exciting source has been removed. This means that the phosphorescent material has the ability to store energy from the radiation and release it gradually at a separate time. In both cases the material is stimulated by a radiation at a certain energy and light of a lower energy is emitted.

Concerning luminescence (true or false)
    a. Luminescence is the process in which a material absorbs energy from an external source and can emit energy as visible light.
    b. The colour of light emitted depends on the amount of energy absorbed.
    c. Luminescence cannot be used for the measurement of radiation dose.
    d. Luminescence occurs in both the input phosphor and the output phosphor of an image intensifier.
    e. Luminescence occurs in amorphous selenium (a-Se) flat panel detectors used in digital radiography.

Answers

a. Luminescence is the process in which a material absorbs energy from an external source and can emit energy as visible light.

True: Luminescence is defined as the emission of light without the application of heat leading to energy being emitted at reduced energy.

b. The colour of light emitted depends on the amount of energy absorbed.

False: The intensity of the emitted light depends on the amount of energy absorbed.

c. Luminescence cannot be used for the measurement of radiation dose.

False: Luminescence is regularly used to measure radiation.

d. Luminescence occurs in both the input phosphor and the output phosphor of an image intensifier.

True: An image intensifier uses a phosphor in both the input window and the output window. X-rays are converted to visible light at the input window, then to electrons at the photocathode and back to light photons at the output window.

e. Luminescence occurs in a-Se flat panel detectors used in digital radiography.

False: a-Se converts incident x-ray photon energy into electric charge which is subsequently read out. The detector in a computed radiography (CR) system uses phosphorescence to store the detected x-ray pattern and releases the energy as light to be read in the CR reader.

Q1.6 Transverse waves

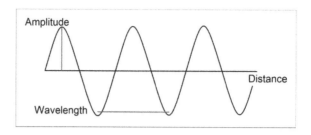

The figure above illustrates a transverse wave and the question challenges your understanding of basic wave properties.

A transverse wave is one where the wave disturbance is perpendicular to the motion of the wave. The amplitude shows the maximum position the wave crest has deviated from the resting position whilst the direction of the wave is at 90° to this.

The frequency of a wave is measured as the number of wave crests that pass a location per unit time, whilst the period of a wave is the reciprocal of the frequency, i.e. the time taken for one wave to pass a fixed point.

One of the interesting things about waves is that they transport energy, not matter or substance. For example, whilst watching waves moving across the sea, you imagine that the water is moving along in the direction of the wave. However, in simple terms the water is moving up and down along the vertical direction as the waves pass through it. The water remains relatively stationary in its overall position in the sea.

Concerning the basic properties of waves (true or false)
    a. Wavelength is defined as the disturbance from an equilibrium position.
    b. Amplitude and intensity are equivalent.
    c. Wave velocity is the product of frequency and wavelength.
    d. The wave period is the reciprocal of the wave frequency.
    e. Longitudinal and transverse waves differ primarily in their direction of displacement relative to the direction of propagation.

Answers
  a. Wavelength is defined as the disturbance from an equilibrium position.
    False: This is the amplitude. The wavelength is the distance between points of equivalent phase. In simple terms this can be considered as the distance between wave peaks or troughs.
  b. Amplitude and intensity are equivalent.
    False: Intensity is proportional (not equivalent) to the square of the amplitude. This therefore means that the intensity cannot be negative, unlike the amplitude which can be negative or positive. The intensity can be considered to be a measure of the effect of the wave.
  c. Wave velocity is the product of frequency and wavelength.
    True: From the equation $v = f \times \lambda$, where $v =$ velocity, $f =$ frequency and $\lambda =$ wavelength. An important aspect of this is to ensure you use the correct units. For instance ensure that you use frequency in Hz rather than MHz and metres instead of centimetres.
  d. The wave period is the reciprocal of the wave frequency.
    True: The frequency is thought of as the number of wave peaks passing a fixed point every second, whereas the period is the time taken for one wavelength to pass the fixed point. Hence the two are related as reciprocals. $T = 1/f$.
  e. Longitudinal and transverse waves differ primarily in their direction of displacement relative to the direction of propagation.
    True: The diagram shows a transverse wave. In a longitudinal wave, the displacement would be such as to reduce or increase the separation between components of the propagating medium.

Q1.7 Longitudinal waves

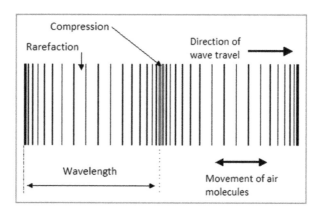

A longitudinal wave is one in which the wave motion is along the direction of propagation. For example, in air the wave consists of areas of compression, where molecules are squeezed together, and rarefaction, where molecules are further apart. This type of wave motion is how ultrasound (US) energy is transmitted through solids, liquids and even gases within the body. The waves obey the laws of physics which govern its transmission and subsequent energy deposition within the tissue, refraction and reflection at tissue boundaries, and scattering within the body.

The constituent particles within the tissue oscillate around a central location much as a spring oscillates around its resting position. This extent of this oscillation is the longitudinal amplitude.

Concerning longitudinal waves (true or false)
    a. A medium is able to transport a wave from one location to another as the particles of the medium interact with each other.
    b. Sound is a longitudinal mechanical pressure wave.
    c. Rarefactions are regions of high pressure.
    d. A sound wave is a series of pressure patterns.
    e. A longitudinal wave may reflect and interfere with other waves at a boundary.

Answers

a. A medium is able to transport a wave from one location to another as the particles of the medium interact with each other.

   True: The medium will be made of molecules or atoms which alter their physical location as the wave passes through the material.

b. Sound is a longitudinal mechanical pressure wave.

   True: A sound wave displaces molecules using areas of compression and rarefaction which indicate areas of high and low pressure.

c. Rarefactions are regions of high pressure.

   False: Areas of rarefaction are low pressure regions.

d. A sound wave is a series of pressure patterns.

   True: There are regular patterns of high and low pressure within the medium.

e. A longitudinal wave may reflect and interfere with other waves at a boundary.

   True: All waves conform to the laws of reflection, refraction and absorption as they pass through media.

Q1.8 The inverse square law

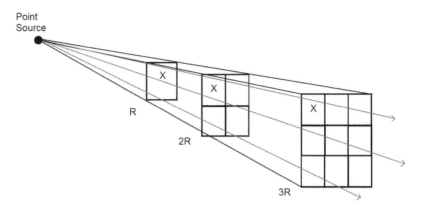

The intensity of radiation emitted from a point source, such as x-rays generated from a focal spot in an x-ray tube (point source in the figure), fall off rapidly the further away you are from the source (distance R). From the figure you can see that for each distance R, the same number of x-ray photons will be distributed across an area (X), then four times the area at $2R$, then nine times the area at $3R$. The number of photons will have reduced by a factor of four, then a factor of nine. Therefore, we say that the number of photons decreases at a rate of the square of the distance from the source—the inverse square law.

Concerning x-rays leaving a point source (true or false)
    a. Doubling the distance reduces the intensity by a factor of four.
    b. Four times the distance reduces the intensity by a factor of 16.
    c. The further away you are from the source the smaller the relative reduction.
    d. Putting distance between staff and a radiation source is a poor method of radiation protection.
    e. An x-ray tube with a large focal spot (1.5 mm × 1.5 mm) does not really obey the inverse square law.

Answers

a. Doubling the distance reduces the intensity by a factor of four.

   True: The inverse square law obeys $1/R^2$ where R is the distance, so doubling the distance from 1 m to 2 m means $1/2^2$ which shows that the radiation intensity will fall by a factor of four.

b. Four times the distance reduces the intensity by a factor of 16.

   True: Put a value of 4 into the equation for R ($1/4^2$) which indicates that the intensity will fall by a factor of 16.

c. The further away you are from the source the smaller the relative reduction.

   True: The following table shows the relative reductions in intensity of an x-ray beam for distances of 1 m, 2 m, 3 m and 4 m.

Distance (metres)	$1/R^2$	Relative reduction
1	1	1
2	1/4	4
3	1/9	2.25
4	1/16	1.778

d. Putting distance between staff and a radiation source is a poor method of radiation protection.

   False: This is an excellent method of reducing radiation intensity, move away as far as possible.

e. An x-ray tube with a large focal spot (1.5 mm × 1.5 mm) does not really obey the inverse square law.

   False: Compared to the distances within an x-ray room, this focal spot is very small and can be considered as a point source.

Q1.9 Radioactivity in medicine

Name	Atomic number	Alpha	Beta	Gamma
Caesium-137	55		X	X
Cobalt-60	27		X	X
Iodine-129 and -131	53		X	X
Radium	88	X		X
Radon	86	X		
Strontium-90	38		X	
Technetium-99	43		X	X
Thorium	90	X		X

Radioactivity is due to the presence of unstable nuclei within isotopes. A stable nucleus is one which contains equal (or nearly equal) numbers of protons and neutrons (with the exception of hydrogen). Heavier nuclei have more neutrons and they tend to be more stable. Radionuclides are unstable elements that transform themselves into stable forms by a combination of alpha, beta and gamma radiation emission from the nucleus. This emission enables the nuclei to lose energy and become more stable. The alpha particle is the same as the helium nucleus and consists of two protons and two neutrons. The beta particle is an electron. A gamma ray is high energy EM radiation.

Concerning radionuclides in medicine (true or false)
   a. The half-life of technetium-99m is 6 days.
   b. Radon is a radioactive gas that is common throughout the natural environment.
   c. Alpha particles only travel a few millimetres in air.
   d. Beta particles can pass through air, paper, aluminium and lead with little attenuation.
   e. Gamma rays are equivalent to x-rays but with higher energy.

Answers

    a. The half-life of technetium-99m is 6 days.

       False: This is a fact to be remembered. A key learning point here is to ensure you look at the units. The actual answer is 6 hours.

    b. Radon is a radioactive gas that is common throughout the natural environment.

       False: This is a misconception. It is a major contributor to dose, but it is actually rare and is usually only commonly found in underground cavities in radon prone areas such as Devon or the Highlands of Scotland.

    c. Alpha particles only travel a few millimetres in air.

       True: Alpha particles are slow and large which increases their chance of being stopped. Air stops them in a centimetre or so and dead skin will also attenuate them, making surface contamination less serious than internal contamination where the alphas may penetrate the digestive tract cell walls and cause damage to the cellular DNA.

    d. Beta particles can pass through air, paper, aluminium and lead with little attenuation.

       False: Although particulate, beta particles are small and fast meaning that they can penetrate many materials. However, although they can penetrate a few metres of air or thin metal such as tin or aluminium, they are stopped by thicker materials and materials such as lead.

    e. Gamma rays are equivalent to x-rays but with higher energy.

       False: This is a subtle difference but EM radiation can have a certain energy but be called something different as a result of its origin. X-rays are created in the electronic orbitals and gammas are from the relaxation of the nucleus.

Q1.10 Radioactive decay

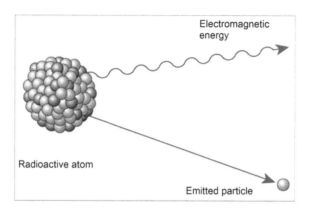

Most nuclei are stable, however, there are some which have an imbalance of neutrons and protons in their nucleus. In order to stabilize, these nuclei release energy from the nucleus in the form of EM radiation (gamma rays) and/or particles, for example, an electron or alpha particle. Radioactive decay is a process that is statistical (stochastic) which means it occurs randomly. We cannot determine when a decay process will occur but for a sample of material we can determine the rate at which radioactive decay occurs (the sample will contain a large number of individual nuclei and therefore the random action may be smoothed out to a certain extent).

The rate of disintegration is known as the activity and is defined as the number of disintegrations per second. The SI unit is the becquerel, where one $Bq = 1$ disintegration per second (s^{-1}).

Concerning radioactive decay (true or false)
- a. A given isotope can only have one type of radiation associated with it.
- b. Atoms with a significant excess of neutrons are likely to be unstable.
- c. Alpha decay involves loss of electrons from the atom.
- d. An atom having undergone a decay is relatively unlikely to undergo a second decay process.
- e. The half-life of an isotope will depend upon the molecular environment in which it is chemically bound.

Answers

a. A given isotope can only have one type of radiation associated with it.

False: Many if not most, isotopes have two or more radioactive pathways. This may be the release of a gamma ray in coincidence with a beta particle. In nuclear medicine, isotopes are selected to have minimal or no secondary radiation since any particulate radiation will only contribute to dose.

b. Atoms with a significant excess of neutrons are likely to be unstable.

True: If there is a large number of neutrons in comparison to protons in the nucleus, this may indicate that the nucleus is unstable and is therefore more likely to decay by the loss of neutrons either by neutron ejection or internal conversion.

c. Alpha decay involves loss of electrons from the atom.

False: Alpha decay is the loss of two neutrons and two protons from the nucleus. Being charged, the loss of the alpha will cause an electron excess. The excess of electrons will then be lost but separately from the alpha release.

d. An atom undergoing a decay to an unstable daughter is relatively unlikely to undergo a second decay process.

False: A radioactive decay event is purely random and hence the same atom is as likely to undergo a second decay. An important point here is that once decay has occurred, then it is a different element and hence the decay path is different from its original form which has a likelihood of decay that is statistically random but it might be different from the original probability of decay.

e. The half-life of an isotope will depend upon the molecular environment in which it is chemically bound.

False: The molecular environment is a chemical consideration which depends on the electron configuration, whereas radioactive decay is a nuclear characteristic.

Q1.11 Exponential decay

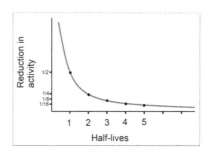

Looking at decay mathematically, we find that the decay process can be described in exponential terms. What this means is that over a fixed period, the half-life, the decay falls to half the original activity, then to one quarter, then to one eighth... This is exponential decay and is common in many natural processes.

$A = A_0 \exp(-k/t)$, where A_0 is the activity at time zero, A is the activity we want to determine after time t and k is a constant for the particular nuclide.

Concerning exponential decay (true or false)
    a. If a radionuclide has an activity of 24 MBq and a half-life of 3 hours, after 9 hours its activity will be 4 MBq.
    b. If a radionuclide has a half-life of 6 hours and its activity is 10 MBq, after 30 hours its activity will have dropped to 1/32 of the original 10 MBq.
    c. The concept of half-life can be applied at any point in time.
    d. The activity of a nuclide never becomes zero.
    e. Physical half-life refers to the reduction in the radioactivity of radionuclides.

Answers

a. If a radionuclide has an activity of 24 MBq and a half-life of 3 hours, after 9 hours its activity will be 4 MBq.

   False: Its decay for each half-life will be as follows, after 3 hours activity will have dropped to 12 MBq, after 6 hours activity will have dropped to 6 MBq and after 9 hours (three half-lives) the activity will be 3 MBq.

b. If a radionuclide has a half-life of 6 hours and its activity is 10 MBq, after 30 hours its activity will have dropped to 1/32 of the original 10 MBq.

   True: After five half-lives, the activity has dropped to 1/32.

c. The concept of half-life can be applied at any point in time.

   True: For any given point in time, after one half-life the activity will be halved.

d. The activity of a nuclide never becomes zero.

   True: As there are billions of nuclei present in a sample and the half-life is finite, the sample can keep halving its activity for a very long time, see the tail on the graph in the figure.

e. Physical half-life refers to the reduction in the radioactivity of radionuclides.

   True: There is a second concept called biological half-life which defines how long the body takes to excrete half the activity.

Q1.12 The half-life of a radionuclide

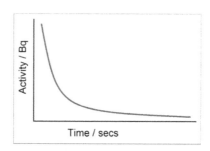

The half-life of a radionuclide is defined as the time taken for its activity to fall to half of its value at first measurement. Therefore, if a radionuclide has an activity of 10 MBq, then after one half-life the remaining activity within the material will be 5 MBq. After five half-lives, the activity would be reduced by 2^5, in this case by a factor of 32, $10/32 = 0.3125$ MBq.

Radioactive decay is a random, unpredictable natural phenomenon. One would imagine that the nuclides that were most unstable would decay the fastest with the shortest half-life, however, this is not the case. The only predictable variable is that the number of nuclei decaying over a short period of time is directly proportional to the number of nuclei present in the sample.

Concerning the half-life of radionuclides (true or false)
  a. The half-life refers to the length of time a radionuclide maintains its radioactivity.
  b. The half-life indicates that radionuclide activity occurs at regular intervals.
  c. The half-life is due to the exponential decay of a radionuclide.
  d. Knowledge of the half-life enables a prediction of which atom is likely to decay.
  e. Large atoms are likely to have long half-lives as a result of the inner nucleons finding it difficult to escape the nucleus.

Answers

a. The half-life refers to the length of time a radionuclide maintains its radioactivity.

  False: The half-life mathematically describes the decay of a radionuclide and is the time taken for the activity of a radionuclide sample to reduce its activity by 50%.

b. The half-life indicates that radionuclide activity occurs at regular intervals.

  False: A radionuclide emits radiation at random and unpredictable times (a stochastic process).

c. The half-life is due to the exponential decay of a radionuclide.

  True: An exponential function describes how the fall of activity of a sample follows a pattern.

d. Knowledge of the half-life enables a prediction of which atom is likely to decay.

  False: The radioactive decay process is purely random.

e. Large atoms are likely to have long half-lives as a result of the inner nucleons finding it difficult to escape the nucleus.

  False: The physical size of the nucleus is not a factor in the half-life. The neutron excess and nuclear energy levels are the primary factors.

Q1.13 Units and measurement

The SI System of Units (Le Système International d'Unités) defines a set of seven base units from which all other units may be generated. These are shown in the table.

Property	Unit name	Symbol
Mass	kilogram	kg
Length	metre	m
Time	second	s
Temperature	kelvin	K
Electric current	ampere	A
Luminosity	candela	cd
Amount of a substance	mole	mol

Other units may be derived from these, for example:
- Density is mass per unit volume (where volume is distance to the power of three) and its unit is $kg\ m^{-3}$.
- Velocity is distance per unit time and therefore its unit is $m\ s^{-1}$.

What are the SI base units for the following measurements?
  a. Blood flow (the unit most often used in US).
  b. Force (in newtons).
  c. Heart rate (beats per minute).
  d. Radioactivity (in becquerels).
  e. Energy (in joules).

Answers
a. Blood flow (the unit most often used in US).
   Distance per unit time = velocity ($m\ s^{-1}$ or $cm\ s^{-1}$).
b. Force (in newtons).
   Force = mass × acceleration ($kg\ m\ s^{-2}$).
c. Heart rate (beats per minute).
   Count per unit time has the unit of s^{-1}.
d. Radioactivity (in becquerels).
   Counts per unit time has the unit of s^{-1}.
e. Energy (in joules).
   Energy = work, where work = force × distance
   Energy = $kg\ m\ s^{-2} \times m = kg\ m^2\ s^{-2}$.

Q1.14 Prefixes to units

In nature and medicine many units have very large ranges associated with them. For example, the dynamic range of measurement of a magnetic resonance (MR) scanner may range from 0 to 10 000 or 20 000, or much higher in specialist machines. Voltages measured within the body for nerve impulse, electrocardiography traces and electroencephalography investigations may range from millionths of volts to a few fractions of a volt. A typical picture archive and communication system may store hundreds of thousands of images per year requiring billions of bytes of computer memory for storage. Therefore we need a range of prefixes that help define these numbers from very small to very large numbers.

Prefix	Number (10^n)	Decimal
nano	10^{-9}	0.000 000 001
micro	10^{-6}	0.000 001
milli	10^{-3}	0.001
centi	10^{-2}	0.01
deci	10^{-1}	0.1
	10^0	1
deca (not common)	10^1	10
hecto (not common)	10^2	100
kilo	10^3	1 000
mega	10^6	1 000 000
giga	10^9	1 000 000 000
tera	10^{12}	1 000 000 000 000

What are the prefixes for the following?
    a. Ferrous based contrast agent in MR.
    b. US frequencies.
    c. MR gradient field strength.
    d. Radiation doses.
    e. Nuclear medicine radionuclide activity.

Answers

    a. nanometres.

    b. MHz.

    c. mT.

    d. mSv.

    e. MBq or GBq.

Q1.15 Full width at half maximum

In mathematics the full width at half maximum (FWHM) is a method to obtain an objective measure of a function that is not clearly defined and does not conform to a geometric structure (e.g. blood vessel diameter, slice thickness, edge definition). It is defined as the cross sectional width of a peak, as shown in the figure, measured at half its maximum height or at 50% of the maximum intensity. In the above figure the peak could be described as having a width of 20 mm (at its base) or about 7 mm around the middle or 4 mm at its peak. FWHM gives us a standard way of measuring the width of a peak in a repeatable fashion.

Concerning FWHM (true or false)
 a. The FWHM can be used to estimate the slice thickness in an MR scanner.
 b. The width of the profile is measured near the maximum intensity region of the profile.
 c. The FWHM is a consideration in assessing the resolving power of an imaging system.
 d. The FWHM is equivalent to the size of the feature being imaged.
 e. The gradient of the sides of the FWHM curve are related to the system modulation transfer function.

Answers

a. The FWHM can be used to estimate the slice thickness in an MR scanner.

   True: The slice profile (sensitivity across the anatomy) is rarely a perfect square shape where the sensitivity is the same across the slice. It is more likely to be a Gaussian or bell shape, and the FWHM is used to get an objective measure of this.

b. The width of the profile is measured near the maximum intensity region of the profile.

   False: The width is measured where the intensity is 50% of the maximum.

c. The FWHM is a consideration in assessing the resolving power of an imaging system.

   True: A system is said to be resolved if the gap between two FWHM curves is clearly visible.

d. The FWHM is equivalent to the size of the feature being imaged.

   False: A poor imaging system will increase the apparent width of the feature being imaged.

e. The gradient of the sides of the FWHM curve are related to the system MTF.

   True: The gradient of the curve sides is steepest when the component spatial frequencies are greatest which is reflected in the cut off frequency of the modulation transfer function.

Q1.16 The point spread function

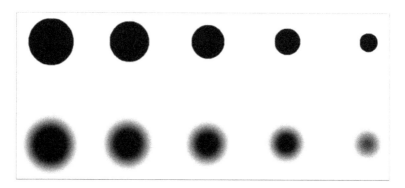

All imaging systems have a tendency to record small high contrast points (or sharp edges) with a degree of blurring. The many reasons for this include multiple steps and technologies in the imaging chain which add inconsistencies, and system noise and distortion to the original signal. This blurring is commonly referred to as the point spread function. In an image a piece of calcified tissue (which has inherent high contrast) may be displayed as a blurred and out of focus object without clear boundaries between it and the surrounding soft tissue.

Concerning the point spread function of an imaging device (true or false)
  a. The point spread function demonstrates how well small objects may be resolved.
  b. Blurring of a point source may not be the same in each direction for an imaging device.
  c. The focal spot size does not affect the point spread function.
  d. Image noise has an impact on the point spread function.
  e. The point spread function is changed by the image reconstruction algorithm.

Answers

a. The point spread function demonstrates how small objects close together may be resolved.

   True: From the figure you can see that the impact of the point spread function is to blur a point source. If two points are close together they may well become merged and unresolved due to this blurring.

b. Blurring of a point source may not be the same in each direction for an imaging device.

   True: This is called an asymmetrical point spread function where the blurring varies with direction around the point source or object.

c. The focal spot size does not affect the point spread function.

   False: The focal spot size of an x-ray imaging system will affect the point spread function, as a large focal spot will cause geometric distortion and therefore blurring of the edges of a sharp object.

d. Image noise has an impact on the point spread function.

   True: The image of a point source may be blurred and degraded due to the presence of noise.

e. The point spread function is changed by the image reconstruction algorithm.

   True: A reconstruction algorithm will have an impact on the edges and sharpness of a point source and may introduce blurring and artefacts which will distort the image. In computed tomography (CT), for example, there are separate bone and soft tissue reconstruction algorithms which give very different appearances to small details in the image (bone algorithms generate images that are usually sharper).

Q1.17 Mathematical considerations

For most applications we do not rely on a precise value of a measurement, but rather estimate a reasonable quantity and from that assess whether a variance from it is significant. For instance, a chest x-ray may impart a dose of 0.01 mSv but that is not significantly different from a dose of 0.011 mSv. An increase of 0.001 mSv may be a 10% elevation in dose but it is not significant to the patient risk.

It is also the case that proportionality is an important concept. At stochastic exposures, risk is proportional to dose but in US risk is not proportional to the mechanical index (MI). MI is a risk indicator which is kept low but is simply used as a method to decrease ultrasonic exposure.

Proportionality, estimation, approximations and simple trend comparators are essential in managing risk and other observations. A question often arising is what constitutes approximate equivalence. If you estimate the height or extent of something, a factor of 10 difference is clearly significant, but a doubling may not be.

From common experience (true or false)
    a. The dose from a chest x-ray is approximately the same as the annual dose from background radiation.
    b. X-ray energy is proportional to wavelength.
    c. The resolution in MR imaging (MRI) is approximately equivalent to that in positron emission tomography (PET).
    d. There is no correlation between Larmor frequency and field strength.
    e. Risk in US increases with thermal index (TI).

Answers

a. The dose from a chest x-ray is approximately the same as the annual dose from background radiation.

False: It is useful to explain to a patient who is concerned about radiation risk that naturally occurring background radiation (2.2 mSv per annum) is approximately a few hundred times larger than the radiation dose due to a chest x-ray (0.01 mSV).

b. X-ray energy is proportional to wavelength.

False: X-ray energy is directly proportional to the radiation frequency and therefore inversely proportional to the wavelength.

c. Resolution in MRI is approximately equivalent to that in PET.

False: The resolution of an MR scanner is approximately 20 line pairs per centimetre (lp cm^{-1}; depending on pixel size) and the spatial resolution of a PET scanner is of the order of 2 lp cm^{-1}.

d. There is no correlation between Larmor frequency and field strength.

False: The Larmor frequency at which protons precess in a strong magnetic field is directly proportional to the field strength. They are related to each other by a constant known as the gyromagnetic frequency, whose units are MHz T^{-1}.

e. Risk in US increases with TI.

True: The TI is the ratio of the power emitted from an US probe to that required to raise the temperature of tissue by 1 °C. Given that heating may have a damaging role in tissue, the greater the TI the greater the risk to tissue. The point to remember here is that the risk increases with TI but is not proportional to it.

Q1.18 Contrast agents I

Contrast agents (media) are routinely used to improve the visibility of anatomical structures or disease within the body. In imaging, the agent is administered orally, rectally, intravenously or intra-arterially, to increase absorption of x-rays, or modify relaxation times according to the selected modality. The contrast media creates a reduced or increased signal on the imaging detector according to the agent used compared to surrounding structures, therefore increasing image contrast. In magnetic resonance imaging the heavy metal element, gadolinium, is chelated with diethylenetriaminetetraacetic acid (DTPA) to form a soluble substance that can be safely administered into the body. The gadolinium complex can become magnetised when placed in an external magnetic field.

Regarding contrast agents in medical imaging (true or false)
  a. Barium is used as a contrast agent in x-ray imaging as it has a low atomic number.
  b. Air may be used as a natural contrast medium.
  c. The absorption edge of iodine enhances its capability of being a contrast medium.
  d. Gadolinium increases the T1 value of tissue to increase image contrast.
  e. Gadolinium demonstrates a strong paramagnetic effect.

Answers

a. Barium is used as a contrast agent in x-ray imaging as it has a low atomic number.

   False: Barium is used as a contrast agent as it has a higher anatomic number (56) compared to both hard (calcium: 20) and soft tissue (< than 8 as oxygen is 65% of the body composition). It produces high contrast due to differential x-ray absorption.

b. Air may be used a natural contrast medium.

   True: Yes, air is introduced as a contrast medium as it is less radio-opaque than surrounding tissues and can be used to displace boundaries thereby making them more visible in complex surroundings.

c. The absorption edge of Iodine enhances its capability of being a contrast medium.

   True: There is a sudden increase in the linear attenuation co-efficient for iodine within the x-ray spectrum, therefore much greater absorption occurs for a large part of the spectrum compared to soft tissue.

d. Gadolinium increases the T1 value of tissue to increase image contrast.

   False: The presence of gadolinium causes T1 to shorten where it is localised and produces an increase in MR signal compared to surrounding tissue where no gadolinium is present.

e. Gadolinium demonstrates a strong paramagnetic effect.

   True: Gadolinium has no inherent ferromagnetic effect but becomes magnetised in the presence of a strong magnetic field.

Q1.19 Contrast agents II

Contrast agents in x-ray imaging vary in osmolarity (solute concentration), viscosity and iodine concentration. Lower osmolarity and viscosity are favoured as lower osmolality is associated with a lower number of adverse events and viscosity plays an important role in the contrast medium delivery. Water based, clear and colourless solutions may be ionic or non-ionic (coupled with an organic compound). In CT imaging, the timing of the scan will be dependent on the tissue type under investigation. If imaging is carried out during the arterial phase of contrast media circulation then blood vessels will be enhanced, however, organs and other tissues will not.

The following are ideal properties of contrast agents in diagnostic imaging (true or false)
   a. Non-toxic.
   b. Should cross the blood-brain barrier.
   c. Easy elimination from the body.
   d. Different physiological properties from blood.
   e. Should be inert when inside the body.

Answers

   a. Non-toxic.

      True: A contrast agent may have some toxicity associated with it, due to its chemical composition, but if it is excreted quickly from the body this will reduce the risk to the patient.

   b. Should cross the blood-brain barrier.

      False: The endothelial cells lining the brain microvasculature prevent circulating chemicals in the body from disrupting neural function.

   c. Easy elimination from the body.

      True: Rapid excretion of a contrast agent reduces the risk of adverse reactions although a rapid breakdown of the contrast agent *in vivo* should also be avoided if the agent is to be of practical use.

   d. Different physiological properties from blood.

      False: If the physiological properties are very different from blood they have the potential to disrupt normal body physiology.

   e. Should be inert when inside the body.

      True: The contrast agent should not chemically react with substances within the body.

IOP Publishing

Scientific Basis of the Royal College of Radiologists Fellowship (2nd Edition)
Illustrated questions and answers
Malcolm Sperrin and John Winder

Chapter 2

X-ray imaging

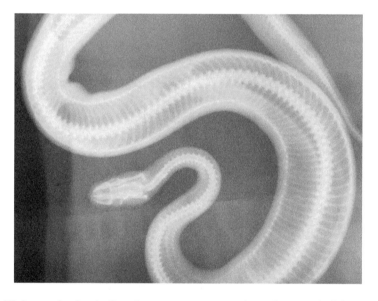

X-rays still form the basis for the most common imaging modalities. Roentgen, in 1895, is attributed with being the original user of X-rays to form an image and it was his 'lucky' wife (Anna Bertha Ludwig Roentgen lived until she was 47 years) whose hand appears on the generally recognised first X-ray generated image. It is a sobering consideration that his wife was therefore one of the earliest recipients of a radiation dose which led in later years to radiation induced damage. X-rays can be used to form images via a number of different methods using projection X-ray, computed tomography, tomography, fluoroscopy, all of which have variations in operation, reconstruction, projection and risk. It is vital

doi:10.1088/978-0-7503-2148-8ch2

to have a full working knowledge of the merits and demerits of each of these. In addition to image formation, you are also expected to be conversant with image contrast, resolution, quality assurance and so on which will inform your clinical decision making processes.

Q2.1 Projection imaging

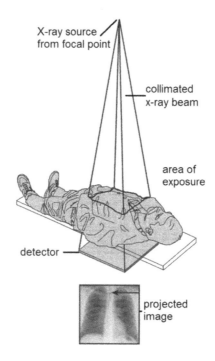

The optical density (OD) of film is defined by the following equation:

$$OD = \log_{10}(\text{incident light/transmitted light}).$$

Note that the measure of OD is logarithmic as this is how the eye responds to the brightness of light (it also converts the transmission into usable numbers). The device to measure this is called a densitometer. If 2% of the light is transmitted through the film then the ratio is 50, thus $OD = \log_{10}(50) = 1.7$, if 1% is transmitted then $OD = \log_{10}(100) = 2.0$. Note that densities with an OD greater than 3.00 are very difficult to see and require a strong light.

Concerning the OD of radiographic film (true or false)
  a. Typical OD ranges from 0.5 to 4.0.
  b. Image contrast is governed by the range of ODs on a film.
  c. OD is increased by the use of an intensifying screen.
  d. Double-sided emulsion does not affect the OD.
  e. OD measures the level of film blackening by passing light through the film.

Answers

a. Typical OD ranges from 0.5 to 4.0.

True: The OD of film is measured by transmitting a known intensity of light through the film and measuring what proportion made it through. The silver grains scatter and absorb the light and the more blackening, the greater the OD.

b. Image contrast is governed by the range of ODs on a film.

True: Image contrast in a radiograph is the difference in OD between two adjacent tissues—if they have the same OD then they have the same blackening and therefore are not separable by viewing and hence there is no contrast between them. The greater the difference in OD between structures the greater the contrast.

c. OD is increased by the use of an intensifying screen.

True: An intensifying screen contains small phosphor grains which absorb x-rays and emit light in proportion to the number of x-rays which has the effect of increasing the sensitivity of the film. For example, a phosphor used in radiography is calcium tungstate which emits blue light after being irradiated with x-rays. Recently, rare earth materials based on lanthanum or gadolinium, which have higher absorption coefficients than calcium tungstate, have been used.

d. Double-sided emulsion does not affect the OD.

False: X-ray film is normally coated on both sides and used in combination with two intensifying screens adjacent to each coating. Each side of the film detector combination absorbs about one third of the x-rays passing through, two thirds in total and therefore increases the blackening and OD.

e. OD measures the level of film blackening by passing light through the film.

True: A densitometer exposes the film to a small (2–3 mm diameter) beam of light that is detected by a photoelectric sensor which measures the amount of light transmitted through the film.

Q2.2 Radiography

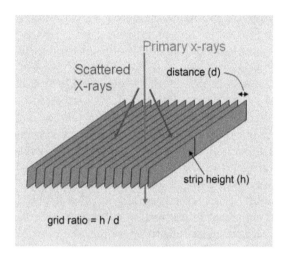

The majority of x-rays projected onto the patient are transmitted directly through to contribute to the overall pattern of x-ray attenuation on the detector and subsequently on the image. However, some x-rays become scattered as they pass through a medium (interactions of x-ray photons with nuclei and electrons). These scattered rays emerge from the patient in random directions and produce a diffuse pattern superimposed onto the actual image. The primary impact of this scattered radiation is to reduce image contrast. One of the ways to overcome this is to use an anti-scatter grid. The grid consists of a series of fine lead strips (less than 0.1 mm thick with a range of 30–80 strips per centimetre).

Concerning the use of anti-scatter grids (true or false)
    a. A grid should always be used to improve image quality.
    b. The grid factor depends on the height and breadth of the collimation spaces.
    c. The grid reduces x-rays coming from scattered radiation.
    d. Grids are normally employed for thin parts of the body like limbs.
    e. Focused grids are used to improve the spatial resolution of the system.

Answers

a. A grid should always be used to improve image quality.

False: Grids are normally used in a wide range of applications where the potential for x-ray scatter and subsequent degradation to image quality is possible. However, scatter reduces with lower kVp and also where the photoelectric effect predominates, e.g. bone imaging.

b. The grid factor depends on the height and breadth of the collimation spaces.

True: The grid factor is calculated as the ratio of the x-ray exposure with the grid to exposure without the grid. This term can be confused with the 'grid ratio (h/d)' which is the ratio of the height of the lead strips (h) to the spacing strip separation (d).

c. The grid reduces x-rays coming from scattered radiation.

True: X-rays that are scattered from the primary beam will traverse at an angle to the beam and become absorbed within the lead strips.

d. Grids are normally employed for thin parts of the body like limbs.

False: Grids are normally used for parts of the body where the x-ray beam has to travel through thicker parts of the body like the head, chest, abdomen and pelvis.

e. Focused grids are used to improve the spatial resolution of the system.

False: A focused grid has its lead strips tilted so that they all point toward the focal spot on the x-ray tube. This enables more of the primary beam to traverse the grid without being absorbed by the lead strips compared to a grid where the leads strips are parallel to each other.

Q2.3 Magnification in radiography

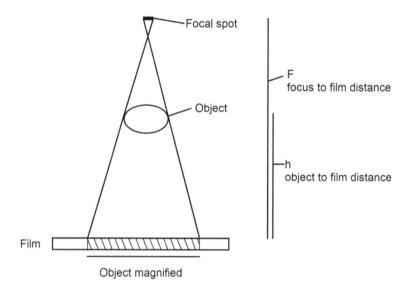

Object magnified

Magnification in radiography is a concept identical to that in normal optics using lenses. It is achieved using different techniques since lenses that focus x-rays are not available but the magnification process is very intuitive as summarized in the figure above.

Concerning magnification in radiography (true or false)
a. Magnification is reduced by using a shorter focus to film distance (FFD).
b. The greater the object to film distance the greater the magnification.
c. Anatomical structures further from the tube focal spot are magnified more.
d. A large focal spot will increase image edge blurring.
e. The penumbra of an image edge can be reduced by using a smaller focal spot.

Answers

a. Magnification is reduced by using a shorter FFD.

False: Magnification (M) is defined as $F/(F - h)$, therefore any increase in F, i.e. the film is moved further away from the object, will result in an increase in magnification. You can demonstrate this using your hand as the object, a light on the ceiling as the source (focal spot) and a table as the detector.

b. The greater the object to film distance the greater the magnification.

True: As the object to film distance is increased the object on the film will be magnified.

c. Anatomical structures further from the tube focal spot are magnified more.

False: For a constant focal spot to film distance, anatomy closer to the focal spot (smaller $F - h$), will be magnified more (greater M).

d. A large focal spot will increase image edge blurring.

True: Blurring at the edge of structures is caused by an increase in focal spot size and is referred to as geometric unsharpness. An infinitely small focal spot would produce a perfectly sharp edge (as shown in the diagram), however, as the focal spot increases in size the projected object edges become blurred (the penumbra).

e. The penumbra of an image edge can be reduced by using a smaller focal spot.

True: This is the opposite of question d, as the focal spot decreases in size, geometric unsharpness decreases and the edges become better delineated, thus reducing the penumbra.

Q2.4 The quality of an x-ray beam

The quality of an x-ray beam is controlled by the voltage applied across the x-ray tube to accelerate the electrons towards the target. An increase in quality is defined as an increase in the mean energy of the x-ray beam. Aluminium filtration improves the quality of the x-ray beam by removing low energy x-ray photons which increases the mean photon energy as shown in the figure. As the mean energy of the beam increases it has more penetrating power. Increasing the mean energy reduces image contrast and decreasing the tube voltage provides more image contrast. However, at low energy there is less penetrating power and more of the beam is absorbed by the subject rather than transmitted through the patient to contribute to the image.

Concerning the x-ray spectrum (true or false)
    a. The higher the tube kV the greater the image contrast.
    b. Increasing kV will give better object penetration and therefore a lower x-ray dose is required for adequate image quality.
    c. Increasing mAs will decrease the signal to noise ratio (SNR).
    d. A larger mA will normally be needed for larger patients.
    e. A combination of mAs and kV is used to control image quality.

Answers

a. The higher the tube kV the greater the image contrast.

False: Although increasing the x-ray tube kV increases the penetrating power of the beam, it also increases the exposure latitude and therefore a larger range of tissues is visualized. This has the impact of reducing overall image contrast.

b. Increasing kV will give better object penetration and therefore a lower x-ray dose is required for adequate image quality.

True: Using a higher kV will result in more energetic x-rays (proportionately more x-rays with a higher kV) which will penetrate the body further and exit to contribute to the image.

c. Increasing mAs will decrease the SNR.

False: An increase in mAs means that the intensity or number of x-rays (n) transmitted to the subject is greater. The noise in the image is proportional to $\sqrt{n}$, and since SNR is $n/\sqrt{n}$, increasing n will result in an increase in SNR. Try putting some values of n into the equation, calculating the SNR and increasing n to see what happens.

d. A larger mA will normally be needed for larger patients.

True: A larger patient will absorb more x-ray photons as the beam traverses the body, therefore a larger mA will provide more x-rays to reach the detector.

e. A combination of mAs and kV is used to control image quality.

True: The kV will affect both SNR and contrast, whilst the mAs will affect the 'brightness' and noise content within the image.

Q2.5 Image quality

Image quality may be defined by three numerical parameters: contrast, spatial resolution and noise. There are many factors that affect these qualities, such as subject contrast, contrast media, x-ray beam quality, subject movement, geometric distortion, scatter radiation and equipment configuration. It should also be remembered that no matter what the image quality, if the image is not fit for purpose, i.e. correct diagnosis or accurate visualization of disease, then it is not useful.

Concerning radiographic image quality (true or false)
  a. A short exposure time will reduce subject movement.
  b. Spatial resolution is unaffected by system unsharpness.
  c. The amount of image noise is unaffected by the patient dose.
  d. Compression of the anatomy increases image contrast and decreases dose.
  e. Image contrast between tissues of high inherent contrast is relatively unaffected by noise.

Answers

a. A short exposure time will reduce subject movement.

True: Subject movement, whether it is breathing, heartbeat, pulsation of tissues due to blood flow or gross movement, will be reduced by a shorter exposure time as there will be less time during image collection for the subject to move.

b. Spatial resolution is unaffected by system unsharpness.

False: Spatial resolution is the ability of an imaging system to differentiate between two objects which are close together, i.e. to resolve them. The system unsharpness may be affected by geometric unsharpness, screen/film unsharpness, pixel size and subject movement.

c. The amount of image noise is unaffected by the patient dose.

False: Patient dose is affected by many parameters including kV, mA, exposure time (s), which is directly related to the number of x-rays delivered.

d. Compression of the anatomy increases image contrast and decreases dose.

True: The use of compression in x-ray imaging creates more uniform tissue thickness, especially across the breast. It makes the tissue thinner which requires a lower dose to penetrate, reducing dose and scattered radiation. Reduction in scatter will increase tissue contrast.

e. Image contrast between tissues of high inherent contrast is relatively unaffected by noise.

True: Soft tissue and air have very high inherent contrast, therefore the impact of noise will be minimal, up to the point at which the noise is so great that it breaks up internal anatomical structure or affects the definition of anatomical edges.

Q2.6 Plain film x-ray tomography

Tomography is central to the use of imaging in medicine. Its aim is to produce a two-dimensional image from the original three-dimensional object without the overlying features contributing to ambiguity as in a plain film x-ray. CT uses back projection to generate the tomographic image but other techniques exist such as tomosynthesis.

Concerning tomosynthesis (true or false)
    a. Geometric unsharpness is exploited to blur images of structures outside the focal plane.
    b. A narrow movement arc creates a thin tomographic section.
    c. The visibility of structures in the focal plane is improved because of increased spatial resolution.
    d. The visibility of structures in the focal plane is improved by reducing the visibility of overlying and underlying structures.
    e. High contrast structures may cause artefacts outside the focal plane.

Answers

a. Geometric unsharpness is exploited to blur images of structures outside the focal plane.

False: If you think about the motion of the x-ray tube and film cassette as they move relative to each other, there is a plane between (aligned with the pivot point or fulcrum) in which structures remain projected onto the same part of the film. The projected image of structures which are above or below this plane moves across the film and becomes blurred. This blurring means they lose contrast and definition and therefore sharpness and good contrast.

b. A narrow movement arc creates a thin tomographic section.

False: The greater the angle of swing or movement of the x-ray tube the thinner the tomographic section.

c. The visibility of structures in the focal plane is improved because of increased spatial resolution.

False: The spatial resolution is defined by factors such as focal spot size, geometric unsharpness and movement.

d. The visibility of structures in the focal plane is improved by reducing the visibility of overlying and underlying structures.

True: The blurring of structures outside the focal plane reduces their visibility.

e. High contrast structures may cause artefacts outside the focal plane.

True: High contrast objects will appear as light or dark streaks on a tomogram and will appear artefactual.

Q2.7 Fluoroscopy technology

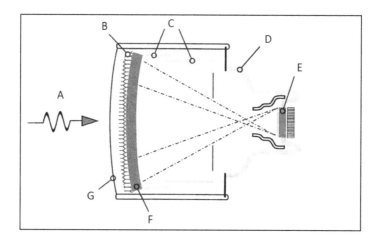

The image above is a schematic of a component used in fluoroscopy. Name the parts of the image intensifier labelled A–G.

Answers

  a. Incident x-ray beam.
  b. Input phosphor.
  c. Focusing electrodes.
  d. Image intensifier housing (ceramic/metal).
  e. Output phosphor.
  f. Photocathode.
  g. Input window.

Q2.8 Image intensifier

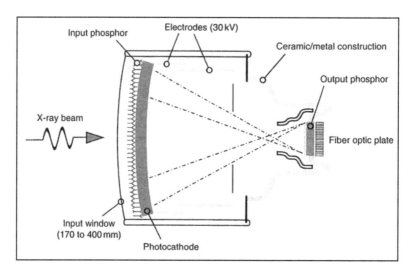

The purpose of an image intensifier in fluoroscopy is to convert a real-time x-ray image into one that can be viewed using visible light. This requires first the detection of x-rays (after passing through the subject) by a phosphor and subsequent conversion of light to electrons through a photocathode surface. The intensity of the light from the input phosphor and subsequent electrons from the photocathode are directly proportional to the intensity of the x-rays. The input screen is curved with a radius that approximates the distance from the subject to create as even an illumination as possible. The input phosphor is caesium iodide and the photocathode is antimony caesium.

In a fluoroscopy image intensifier (true or false)
   a. A curved input screen is used to match the x-ray focal spot distance.
   b. Caesium iodide is chosen as the input phosphor as it is an efficient convertor of x-rays to light.
   c. The narrow needle-like crystals decrease spatial resolution.
   d. The output screen is about 100 mm in diameter.
   e. The output screen has an anode which is a phosphor layer with a metal coating on one side.

Answers

a. A curved input screen is used to match the x-ray focal spot distance.

False: The curved input screen has a radius of curvature to match the distance from the input screen to the focal point of the electron beam at the other end of the intensifier.

b. Caesium iodide is chosen as the input phosphor as it is an efficient convertor of x-rays to light.

True: The phosphor layer is invariably caesium iodide which captures about 60% of the x-rays incident upon it.

c. The narrow needle-like crystals decrease spatial resolution.

False: The purpose of the caesium iodide needle-shaped crystals is to improve spatial resolution as the needle structure acts a light guide using internal reflection to minimize the spread of the light.

d. The output screen is about 100 mm in diameter.

False: The output screen is typically 25–30 mm in diameter.

e. The output screen has an anode which is a phosphor layer with a metal coating on one side.

True: The metal coating on the inside of the output screen phosphor acts as an anode and also as a backing to the phosphor layer to prevent light back-scattering onto the input phosphor which would subsequently cause an avalanche of electrons.

Q2.9 Fluoroscopy radiation dose

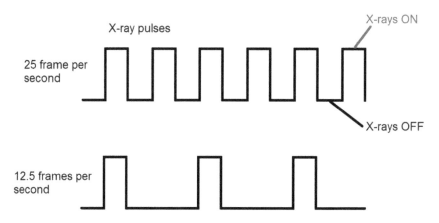

Radiation dose in fluoroscopy is dependent on a range of factors (apart from mA, kV, tube distance and filtration) including the overall screening time, the efficiency of the image intensifier, the x-ray pulse rate and the expertise of the operator. Dose rate can be reduced significantly using the simple control of the x-ray pulse rate whereby halving the pulse approximately halves the dose. Frame rates of up to 30 frames per second (fps) may be used and these appear on the screen as continuous images as the eye cannot detect the individual frames.

Concerning dose control in fluoroscopy (true or false)
    a. Dose is maintained by a feedback system from the television brightness linked to the kV and mA of the x-ray tube.
    b. Dose control is achieved by minimizing the pulse rate of the system at all times.
    c. The dose rate can be roughly halved by changing from a frame rate of 25 fps to 12.5 fps.
    d. Dose may be controlled by the automatic gain control system.
    e. Dose is partly dependent on the time taken for the imaging investigation.

Answers

a. Dose is maintained by a feedback system from the television brightness linked to the kV and mA of the x-ray tube.

   True: In optical systems a small sample of the light generated at the output phosphor is sampled using a mirror system and the kV and mAs adjusted accordingly.

b. Dose control is achieved by minimizing the pulse rate of the system at all times.

   False: Minimizing the frame rate (say to one per second) would have a very adverse effect on the smoothness and appearance of the 'live' image on screen, the lower the frame rate the more lag or blurring would be apparent.

c. The dose rate can be roughly halved by changing from a frame rate of 25 fps to 12.5 fps.

   True: For each frame the x-ray pulse size will remain the same to ensure correct exposure, however, the rate at which the pulses are delivered will have a direct impact on the dose rate.

d. Dose may be controlled by the automatic gain control system.

   True: In this case the automatic gain control is that of the television system, so that if kV and mA were not altered for a change in patient (radiological) thickness, the brightness of the television could be controlled by its gain setting.

e. Dose is partly dependent on the time taken for the imaging investigation.

   True: Radiation doses in fluoroscopy are due to screening times and direct exposures to generate images. Therefore a procedure that requires a longer screening time will affect the overall examination dose.

Q2.10 Image quality in fluoroscopy

A fluoroscopy system contains a complex chain of technology which is linked by various detectors and transducers, where different energy forms are converted from one to another. Each step in the chain affects image quality, usually to its detriment. The chain consists of an input screen (phosphor) which detects x-rays and a photocathode with a needle like crystal structure. This structure helps prevent the scatter of light within the photocathode. Electrons accelerated by 25 kV impact on the output screen which converts their energy into visible light that is picked up and displayed by a television system.

In a fluoroscopy system (true or false)
a. The spatial resolution of the intensifier is typically 4–5 line pairs per millimetre (lp mm^{-1}).
b. The television system or charge-coupled device (CCD) camera may degrade the image quality.
c. The narrow needle-like crystals in the input phosphor are made of BGO (bismuth germinate orthophosphate).
d. Noise may be reduced by increasing the CCD camera gain.
e. Stray light inside the image intensifier may increase image contrast.

Answers

a. The spatial resolution of the intensifier is typically 4–5 lp mm^{-1}.

True: Spatial resolution is limited by blurring due to the output phosphor and can be increased using magnification techniques.

b. The television system or CCD camera may degrade the image quality.

True: The image display on the monitor is generally less that 4–5 lp mm^{-1} as the television system or CCD camera degrade the image due to their weaker resolving power.

c. The narrow needle-like crystals in the input phosphor are made of 'BGO'.

False: They are made of CSI doped with Na.

d. Noise may be reduced by increasing the CCD camera gain.

False: The limit to the noise level in an image intensifier is the number of x-ray photons impinging on the input phosphor, therefore no adjustments to settings after this point will change the noise levels.

e. Stray light inside the image intensifier may increase image contrast.

False: The impact of stray light within the image intensifier, which may result from output phosphor, electron or x-ray scatter within the housing, will reduce the overall image contrast in the same way as it does for conventional radiographic imaging.

Q2.11 High kV technique

Image contrast in conventional x-ray imaging is controlled primarily by the x-ray tube kV. The kV setting will control both the quality and quantity of x-ray photons. For greater kV, the x-rays penetrate tissues more uniformly with a variety of densities. For example, in a chest x-ray there is very high inherent contrast between the main components of the chest, for example, bone, lung, air, muscle, etc; a reduction in contrast results in a more useful image. Low kV would result in very high contrast between the ribs and the lungs, potentially obscuring details. A high kV setting is typically 120–140 kV.

Concerning the use of the high kV technique (true or false)
   a. The technique usually results in a reduction in radiographic contrast.
   b. An air gap technique may be used.
   c. The technique usually results in increased patient dose.
   d. The technique can be used to obtain better visualization of bone lesions.
   e. The technique usually improves the visualization of lesions in the breast.

Answers

a. The technique usually results in a reduction in radiographic contrast.

True: The purpose of high kV in the chest is to reduce inherent contrast between bone, soft tissue and air filled tissue.

b. An air gap technique may be used.

True: An air gap technique may be used as the high kV setting increases forward scatter but there is sufficient sideways scatter for this to be useful.

c. The technique usually results in increased patient dose.

False: A decreased radiation dose should be experienced with a high kV technique.

d. The technique can be used to obtain better visualization of bone lesions.

False: Bone lesions require high contrast to discriminate between tissues of similar attenuation coefficients. Increasing kV reduces the attenuation coefficient difference and hence decreases resolution.

e. The technique usually improves the visualization of lesions in the breast.

False: The attenuation coefficient variation between soft tissues is small and hence any technique designed to identify the location of such tissue must be able to utilize what contrast is available. As kV increases, the linear attenuation coefficient for soft tissue approximates to the same value and hence contrast is lost making low kV the preferred technique in mammography.

Q2.12 Mammography x-ray spectra

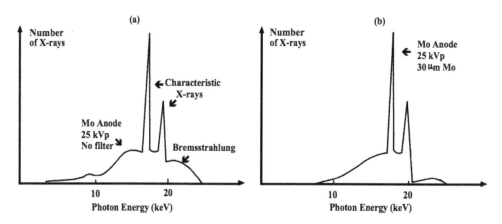

The x-ray spectrum for a mammography set is a combination of bremsstrahlung and characteristic radiation. A molybdenum target produces the x-ray spectrum in figure (a) and a molybdenum filter is used in the equipment to remove low energy (or soft) x-rays below 20 keV and also bremsstrahlung above the characteristic x-rays in figure (b). The purpose of this is to reduce the radiation exposure to the breast whilst maintaining the strength of characteristic x-rays which contribute strongly to the image. Thicker breasts require slightly higher mean energy within the x-ray beam and therefore an alloy of molybdenum and rhodium or pure rhodium is used.

In mammography (true or false)

    a. K-edges are regions in the x-ray spectrum where there is preferential absorption.

    b. Reduction in tube kVp will increase image contrast at the expense of dose.

    c. Characteristic radiation at 17.9 and 19.6 keV is used to improve image contrast.

    d. A molybdenum window is used to reduce radiation dose to the breast.

    e. The k-edges of the x-ray spectrum are increased proportionately by using a molybdenum window.

Answers

a. K-edges are regions in the x-ray spectrum where there is preferential absorption.

   True: K-edges are produced where the x-ray energy of incident photons is just greater than the binding energy of k-shell electrons and gives rise to an increase in the x-ray attenuation.

b. Reduction in tube kVp will increase image contrast at the expense of dose.

   False: Mammography uses a much lower kVp than traditional CR/direct radiography (DR) systems to improve inherent tissue contrast between tissues of very similar x-ray characteristics.

c. Characteristic radiation at 17.9 and 19.6 keV is used to improve image contrast.

   True: These two characteristic radiation peaks are close to the optimum for breast imaging and by strengthening these (removing bremsstrahlung radiation above and below these peaks) will improve image contrast.

d. A molybdenum window is used to reduce radiation dose to the breast.

   True: Molybdenum substantially reduces radiation below 20 keV which would mostly be absorbed by the tissues of the breast and only contribute to patient dose.

e. The k-edges of the x-ray spectrum are increased proportionately by using a molybdenum window.

   True: The purpose of filtration is to remove low energy radiation from the x-ray spectrum and enhance the proportion of x-rays that contribute to the overall image quality (in this case the k-edges).

Q2.13 Mammography spatial resolution

X-ray mammography requires very high spatial resolution compared to conventional x-ray imaging of other parts of the body and the detector should be of the order of 24×30 cm to capture the whole of the breast. One of the main anatomical features it is trying to detect is the presence of tiny deposits of calcification which give an indication of malignancy. Compton scatter results in blurring of the image due to scattered photons being deposited elsewhere within the body. This can partly be reduced by pre-processing of the digital image. Also, lower contrast structural features of the breast are important in detecting changes that are characteristic of breast cancer, therefore high soft tissue contrast is also required.

Concerning x-ray mammography spatial resolution (true or false)
  a. A thin single sided screen is used to help improve spatial resolution.
  b. The small focal spot size used for magnification is typically 0.4 mm.
  c. The typical spatial resolution is usually of the order of 15 lp mm^{-1}.
  d. Mammography requires high spatial resolution to detect low contrast tissue differences.
  e. Overall image sharpness is improved by breast compression.

Answers

a. A thin single sided screen is used to help improve spatial resolution.

   True: Single sided emulsions are used in mammography film as the double sided (thicker) films allow for scatter between the two detecting surfaces and introduce a level of blurring.

b. The small focal spot size used for magnification is typically 0.4 mm.

   False: A 0.4 mm focal spot size is typically used for standard views, a magnified view will use a focal spot size of 0.1 mm.

c. The typical spatial resolution is usually of the order of 15 lp mm^{-1}.

   True: Due to the need to detect microcalcification (down to 100 μm) within the breast tissue a high spatial resolution is required.

d. Mammography requires high spatial resolution to detect low contrast tissue differences.

   False: High spatial resolution is required to detect small high contrast objects, such as calcification, high contrast resolution is required to detect small differences in tissue density.

e. Overall image sharpness is improved by breast compression.

   True: Breast compression is performed to a force of 100–150 newtons (N), this will reduce the breast tissue depth and reduce the degree of scatter. Both spatial resolution (due to reduction in motion and geometric unsharpness) and image contrast (due to separation of superimposed tissues) are improved by this method.

Q2.14 Image quality in mammography

Image quality in mammography is dependent on a number of factors. Contrast is required between soft tissues and also for microcalcification, therefore a low kV technique is used along with high spatial resolution. A very small focal spot size is used (0.3–0.4 mm) to reduce geometric distortion and blurring. The anode heel effect is utilized with the more intense part of the beam transmitted through the breast at the chest wall where the breast is generally thicker, thus providing a better uniformity to images.

Concerning image quality in mammography (true or false)
  a. Compression reduces movement, geometric unsharpness and scattered radiation.
  b. The anode heel effect is positioned to coincide with the nipple edge of the breast.
  c. Compression creates a more homogeneous density across the image.
  d. Movement is not a problem due to short exposure times.
  e. A moving grid is used to reduce scatter.

Answers

a. Compression reduces movement, geometric unsharpness and scattered radiation.
   True: The compression of the breast during mammography holds the soft tissue firmly to reduce movement and make the breast thinner which subsequently reduces geometric unsharpness and reduces scatter as the path length of x-rays is shorter.

b. The anode heel effect is positioned to coincide with the nipple edge of the breast.
   False: The anode heel effect causes a reduction in x-ray beam output on the tube cathode side due to the extra path that x-rays need to travel through the target material. Therefore the more intense part of the beam (anode side) is directed through the chest wall and the less intense part through the nipple side of the breast.

c. Compression creates a more homogeneous density across the image.
   True: Compression causes breast tissue to be more uniformly constant in thickness by spreading it over a wider area which will help to improve image uniformity.

d. Movement is not a problem due to short exposure times.
   False: Exposure times in mammography are long at around 2 s, therefore compression helps to reduce movement.

e. A moving grid is used to reduce scatter.
   True: A moving grid is used in mammography to reduce scatter. The movement of the grid is possible in mammography because of the relatively long exposure times which makes the grid lines much less apparent on the image.

Q2.15 Mammography technology

The mammographic system differs from conventional x-ray systems in some small ways. The x-ray tube operates at a lower kVp, the anode target and filtration are of a different material, and a compression plate is used to compress the breast into an even thickness.

Concerning x-ray mammography technology (true or false)
   a. A typical digital mammography image matrix is 1024×1024 pixels.
   b. The active area of the detector is around 45×34 cm.
   c. The most common target material in mammography systems is rhodium.
   d. Rhodium targets are used in combination with molybdenum for thicker breast tissue in mammography.
   e. Screens are thinner in mammography compared to conventional radiography.

Answers

a. A typical mammography digital image matrix is 1024×1024 pixels.

False: Digital mammography detectors produce very high resolution images with an image matrix of around 5000×4000 pixels.

b. The active area of the detector is around 45×34 cm.

False: A typical mammography digital image detector has an active area in the range 18×23 to 24×30 cm.

c. The most common target material in mammography systems is rhodium.

False: The most common material used in mammography is molybdenum.

d. Rhodium targets are used in combination with molybdenum for thicker breast tissue in mammography.

True: Rhodium is used in the target and filter to produce characteristic radiation at a slightly higher energy than molybdenum which penetrates tissue better.

e. Screens are thinner in mammography compared to conventional radiography.

True: A single screen is used with a single emulsion film to produce a thinner detector and therefore less screen unsharpness.

Q2.16 Mammography compression

Compressing the breast for imaging has an impact in a number of areas. Making the breast thinner means there is less tissue to traverse and therefore fewer x-rays are required. In addition to this, reducing the thickness of the breast reduces the amount of x-ray scatter and therefore improves image quality. Holding the breast still during the examination reduces the potential for subject movement and any subsequent blurring.

Concerning compression in mammography (true or false)
    a. Compression reduces the radiation dose to the breast.
    b. The primary purpose is to reduce the thickness of irradiated tissue.
    c. The amount of compression can be reduced in digital mammography.
    d. Compression reduces scatter.
    e. Compression must be less than 50 N.

Answers

a. Compression reduces the radiation dose to the breast.

True: Compression of the breast, although applied with the same force to all women, will provide a significant thinning of the tissue to approximately the same thickness. This reduces the amount of x-rays required to traverse the breast and also reduces scatter.

b. The primary purpose is to reduce the thickness of irradiated tissue.

True: Thinning the tissue has the impact of dose reduction, however, the breast is also held firmly by the compression plates which helps reduce motion artefacts.

c. The amount of compression can be reduced in digital mammography.

False: If compression is reduced then scatter will likely increase and research has shown that greater compression improves digital mammography image quality.

d. Compression reduces scatter.

True: As the tissue is thinned to around 4 cm the amount of scattered radiation is reduced.

e. Compression must be less than 50 N.

False: The compression forces required in mammography are larger than this for both craniocaudal and mediolateral oblique views. Typical forces range from 70 to 140 N.

Q2.17 Digital mammography

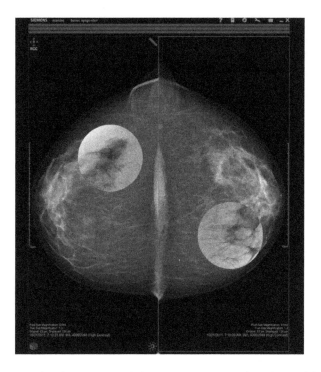

Digital mammography has emerged in recent years with the ability to produce images of comparable diagnostic quality to previous film based systems. It has replaced many film based systems and has better contrast resolution and a greater dynamic range. Although it has poorer spatial resolution, it results in fewer over-exposures. Digital systems have enabled post processing and rapid transfer of images for second reading and computer assisted diagnosis.

Concerning digital mammography (true or false)
  a. The dynamic range is increased in digital systems.
  b. Spatial resolution is improved compared with analogue mammography.
  c. The detector material is often sodium iodide.
  d. Tomosynthesis requires the same radiation dose as standard digital mammography.
  e. The dose is generally lower than that of analogue mammography.

Answers

a. The dynamic range is increased in digital systems.

   True: The dynamic range of digital systems is higher than that of film based systems.

b. Spatial resolution is improved compared with analogue mammography.

   False: Film based spatial resolution is of the order of 17–$10\,\mathrm{lp}\ \mathrm{mm}^{-1}$ whilst digital systems have a spatial resolution of 5–$10\,\mathrm{lp}\ \mathrm{mm}^{-1}$.

c. The detector material is often sodium iodide.

   False: The detector is typically caesium iodide or more recently amorphous selenium (a-Se) and follows CR and DR in their configuration of detector usage.

d. Tomosynthesis requires the same radiation dose as standard digital mammography.

   False: Breast tomosynthesis produces three-dimensional mammograms, however, it requires higher amounts of radiation to achieve useful images.

e. The dose is generally lower than that of analogue mammography.

   True: A recent trial in the US demonstrated that digital mammography can deliver a radiation dose saving of up to 22%.

Q2.18 Computed radiography I

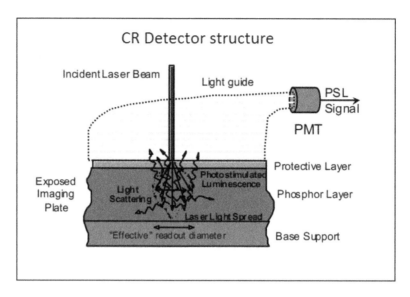

Traditional image capture required the use of acetate and wet chemistry which was bulky, time consuming and presented a risk of fire. The advent of modern semi-conductors and the miniaturization of electronics made the use of solid state detectors possible and this permitted a revolution in image capture. There are many advantages of CR techniques that relate to dose, immediacy, etc, as well as some that relate to cost, all of which are discussed in the key literature.

Concerning detectors in CR (true or false)
    a. The detector releases light in proportion to the incident x-ray intensity.
    b. The storage phosphor is called photostimulable as it detects x-rays.
    c. The detector must be erased before being used for a new exposure.
    d. The detector is 'read' using a CCD camera.
    e. The typical spatial resolution is better than that of conventional film-screen radiography.

Answers

a. The detector releases light in proportion to the incident x-ray intensity.

True: DR uses a storage phosphor that can release energy previously trapped due to incident x-rays and the intensity of light released is proportional to the incident x-ray intensity.

b. The storage phosphor is called photostimulable as it detects x-rays.

True: A laser is used to stimulate the phosphor which causes electrons to relax to lower energy levels, releasing light in the process.

c. The detector must be erased before being used for a new exposure.

True: After stimulation by laser light the whole CR plate is exposed to red LEDs which stimulate any residual charge and further light is released, resulting in the plate being erased for use again.

d. The detector is 'read' using a CCD camera.

False: The detector (plate) is read by illuminating the surface with a laser and the resulting light output is measured by a photomultiplier (PM).

e. The typical spatial resolution is better than that of conventional film-screen radiography.

False: Typically, spatial resolution for a CR image is less than that of a conventional film based x-ray. The pixel size is the governing factor and can vary with plate size. It ranges from 3.5 to 5.5 lp mm^{-1} for a CR image, whereas spatial resolution for a film–screen combination is 8–12 lp mm^{-1}.

Q2.19 Computed radiography II

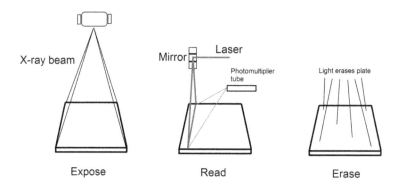

Any imaging process has a degrading effect on the quality of the original object. The type of detector, how it is used and subsequent storage and display are all factors in determining the final image quality. A lot of time, effort and, inevitably, cost is spent in ensuring that each stage of the imaging process is neither a retrograde step nor makes the image of dubious image quality.

Concerning CR image quality (true or false)
    a. The pixel size is determined only by the diameter of the laser beam.
    b. The image pixel size is the limit to spatial resolution.
    c. Larger detectors have lower spatial resolution than small detectors.
    d. The impact of ghost images is reduced by erasing the CR plate.
    e. Dead pixels are filled in by an algorithm.

Answers

a. The pixel size is determined only by the diameter of the laser beam.

False: The pixel size in CR is determined by the timing (clocking speed) of the PM tube as it digitizes the light signal emitted rather than the laser beam diameter.

b. The image pixel size is the limit to spatial resolution.

False: The factors that affect the spatial resolution of a CR imaging system are pixel size, scattered laser light within the imaging plate, the size of the phosphor grains and the diameter of the read-out laser beam.

c. Larger detectors have lower spatial resolution than small detectors.

True: Manufacturers have changed the size of the image matrix obtained with a small plate compared to a large plate (for the chest) as it is thought that the full details obtained by smaller plate imaging are not required for larger fields of view (FOV).

d. The impact of ghost images is reduced by erasing the CR plate.

True: A ghost image is due to residual charge remaining on a CR plate that has already been read, but not erased using a strong red light source.

e. Dead pixels are filled in by an algorithm.

True: A dead pixel is one that contains no usable data and may look black or white on the screen. It can be filled with data using neighbouring pixel data.

Q2.20 Computed radiography: dynamic range

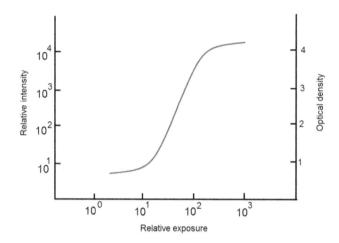

The dynamic range of an imaging system describes the range of signals (from minimum to maximum) that it is able to detect. This means that the system can detect x-ray photons in the range from 10 to around 10 000 (10^4). As a much greater range of exposures can be visualized with image processing, images can be presented even if under- or overexposed. These data would have been lost using conventional film and a repeat x-ray would have been required.

The dynamic range of a CR system (true or false)
    a. Relates to the quantum mottle within the image.
    b. Determines the range of x-ray intensities detected.
    c. Is about 100 : 1.
    d. Is less than that of a conventional film–screen system.
    e. Can cope with a very wide range of x-ray intensities.

Answers

a. Relates to the quantum mottle within the image.

False: Quantum mottle refers to the variation in grey level intensity due to the quantum nature of the detection of x-rays. This means that an area (tissue) of uniform intensity has subtle but visible variation in the apparent density.

b. Determines the range of x-ray intensities detected.

True: The dynamic range of an imaging system refers to the range of x-ray intensity that is detectable from the minimum intensity to the maximum, usually lying on a linear portion of a response curve.

c. Is about 100 : 1.

False: The dynamic range of a CR system is 10 000 : 1.

d. Is less than that of a conventional film–screen system.

False: The dynamic range of a film–screen combination is much lower and non-linear compared to a digital system.

e. Can cope with a very wide range of x-ray intensities.

True: Due to the large dynamic range of CR the system can cope with a wide range of x-ray intensities.

Q2.21 Computed radiography cassettes

The detector in CR is a photostimulable phosphor, also referred to as the storage phosphor. It is typically made of powdered barium fluorohalide which contains small amounts of europium as a doping agent to increase sensitivity. This powder is mixed with a resin and laid down as a 0.3 mm thick coating onto a conductive layer which is in turn laid on a support layer and laminate. This material absorbs incident x-rays and by doing so promotes electrons to higher energy levels within the material structure. To release this energy as light, the intensity of which is proportional to the number of x-rays incident, the phosphor is exposed to a red laser and the light output is measured.

Concerning CR plates (true or false)
  a. Electrons are stimulated to a higher energy state by x-rays.
  b. UV radiation is used to read the image from the cassette.
  c. Dual phosphor layers are used to enhance the sensitivity of the detector.
  d. Crystals that have aligned structures produces poorer resolution than randomly oriented crystals.
  e. CR plates are time sensitive in that they must be read quickly.

Answers

a. Electrons are stimulated to a higher energy state by x-rays.

True: Due to the structure of the barium fluorohalide crystals, a number of electrons become trapped after exposure to x-rays. These traps are also referred to as higher energy states as incident radiation is required to release them so they can return to their normal state and release light (blue) at the same time.

b. UV radiation is used to read the image from the cassette.

False: The energy required to release the electrons from their traps is in the red/IR region of the EM spectrum.

c. Dual phosphor layers are used to enhance the sensitivity of the detector.

True: A second phosphor layer may also be present requiring a transparent support layer so that the cassette plate may be read from the front and the rear.

d. Crystals that have aligned structures produces poorer resolution than randomly oriented crystals.

False: CR plates that have aligned structures are also referred to as columnar phosphors and allow the light to be channelled out of the phosphor with little lateral spread, thus maintaining spatial resolution.

e. CR plates are time sensitive in that they must be read quickly.

True: CR plates lose their signal over time through a process called spontaneous phosphorescence, caused by thermal energy, therefore it is important to read the plate within a few minutes of x-ray exposure.

Q2.22 Computed radiography detection process

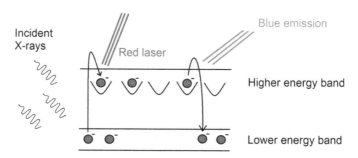

The photostimulable phosphor used in CR imaging is barium fluorohalide (where the halide is a mixture of iodine and bromine). Europium is added as a doping agent which helps to create structures within the crystal lattice that can trap electrons and make the phosphor more sensitive. When exposed to x-rays electrons are moved from a low energy state into a higher energy state where they become trapped. This is where a latent image is stored. It is 'read' by stimulating the electrons using red/IR energy and as the electrons move back to the lower energy state they emit light in the blue region of the visible spectrum.

Concerning photostimulable phosphor (true or false)
   a. One incident photon leads to one excited electron.
   b. The use of a red laser is simply based on cost considerations.
   c. The dopant in the crystal lattice increases the efficiency of the detector.
   d. UV light can also cause excitation of the electrons.
   e. The image is fully erased at the end of the read-out process.

Answers

a. One incident photon leads to one excited electron.

  False: The process is not 100% efficient and the detector efficiency is one factor in considering how the system is optimized. There is a drive to increase the efficiency of the capture process since if more of the x-rays are captured, then the efficiency increases and the dose to the patient can be reduced.

b. The use of a red laser is simply based on cost considerations.

  False: The colour of a laser indicates the energy of the photons. Changing the colour to a longer wavelength will reduce the energy and may be insufficient to cause the excited electrons to decay to their ground state. Decreasing the wavelength will increase the photon energy and will have no benefit but may have sufficient energy to either cause damage or induce further electronic excitement. Cost may be an issue but the physical principles behind the technique are the primary drivers.

c. The dopant in the crystal lattice increases the efficiency of the detector.

  True: The energy levels that are created by the addition of the dopant makes the excited electrons stable for a workable lifetime. Different dopants will reduce the lifetime or make the energy levels inappropriate for use at diagnostic energies.

d. UV light can also cause excitation of the electrons.

  False: The dopant is chosen to ensure that photons of a given energy are absorbed. If this were not the case problems may exist with environmental excitation leading to noise, poor performance, etc.

e. The image is fully erased at the end of the read-out process.

  False: The read-out process is not 100% efficient and it is possible for some electrons to remain in excited states leaving a latent image.

Q2.23 Direct (digital) radiography

An alternative to CR is DR where, whilst still being solid state in nature, the mechanism for obtaining the image is different. Rather than using photo-stimulation, electronic devices are used which change characteristics upon irradiation. There are numerous pros and cons between DR and CR and an understanding of the underlying physics is important in deriving an informed opinion on their use.

Concerning detectors in DR (true or false)
   a. The charge stored in a direct panel detector is directly proportional to the x-ray intensity.
   b. The pixels match the transistors in the array.
   c. In an indirect flat panel detector, elongated caesium iodide crystals greater than the pixel size are used.
   d. The difference between indirect and direct conversion radiography is that one uses amorphous silicon (a-Si) to collect x-rays and the other uses a-Se.
   e. A key advantage over CR is the lower cost of DR.

Answers
a. The charge stored in a direct panel detector is directly proportional to the x-ray intensity.

   True: When x-rays impact on an a-Se detector an electrical charge is generated which is collected by a capacitor and thin film transistor, the greater the x-ray intensity the greater the charge produced.

b. The pixels match the transistors in the array.

   True: After a charge is generated in the a-Se, a thin film transistor array (photodiode array) is used to collect these charges. Each individual transistor is around 100–200 μm, which corresponds to each pixel in the image.

c. In an indirect flat panel detector, elongated caesium iodide crystals greater than the pixel size are used.

   False: The diameters of the caesium iodide crystals are much smaller than the pixel size (thin film transistor) in the detector. This means that light generated due to the interaction of incident x-rays is emitted directly onto the photodiode element by internal reflection.

d. The difference between indirect and direct conversion radiography is that one uses s-Si to collect x-rays and the other uses a-Se.

   False: The indirect capture method captures the x-rays with a caesium iodide crystal and the direct method uses a-Se. Both systems use a silicon based thin film transistor and capacitor configuration to collect an electric charge which is proportional to the amount of incident x-ray photons.

e. A key advantage over CR is the lower cost of DR.

   False: DR detectors are inherently more expensive than CR detectors and much less versatile. Two different detectors would be needed for different bucky positions, whereas there are a wide variety of CR detectors that can easily be placed near the anatomy of interest.

Q2.24 Detectors in direct radiography

The performance of DR and CR detectors is clearly crucial to their effective use in imaging. The physical principles of their design and of the materials used are limiting factors on their use and a knowledge of concepts such as efficiency and sensitivity are crucial.

Concerning detectors in DR (true or false)
  a. The detector quantum efficiency (DQE) depends only on detector efficiency.
  b. The DQE for a DR system may be as high as 90%.
  c. DR systems provide a higher DQE that CR systems.
  d. DR detectors are equally flexible in usage compared to CR cassettes.
  e. DR systems provide a wide dynamic range of x-ray detection.

Answers
a. The DQE depends only on detector efficiency.

   True: The DQE can be conveniently thought of as how close the given detector is to an ideal detector. There are many factors that affect the efficiency of the detector itself but the DQE takes these into account.

b. The DQE for a DR system may be as high as 90%.

   False: The DQE is typically around 60%, although the actual value will vary with photon energy, detector characteristics, etc.

c. DR systems provide a higher DQE that CR systems.

   True: This is simply a fact and the underlying reasons for it relate to the efficiency of the detection process.

d. DR detectors are equally flexible in usage compared to CR cassettes.

   False: CR is essentially a two stage process requiring the cassette to be read out by use of a second stage involving the laser. The DR system can be directly interrogated electronically, making it's use more flexible and less prone to error.

e. DR systems provide a wide dynamic range of x-ray detection.

   True: The dynamic ranges of CR and DR are greater than that for film. Whilst this means that a given patient may receive a slightly higher dose, it also means that there is a reduced need for a repeat exposure following over- or underexposure of the patient. This has the consequence of reducing the population dose.

Q2.25 Breast tomosynthesis

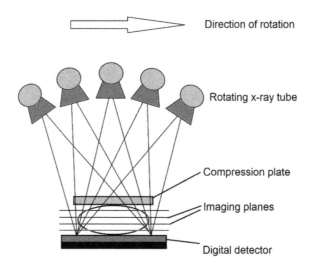

Breast tomosynthesis, which is also referred to as 3D mammography, is a newly emerging technique for the acquisition of volumetric data of the breast. A mammography x-ray tube rotates over the breast in a limited arc, collecting images at regular intervals on a digital detector. It may use continuous acquisition or a 'step and shoot' acquisition depending on the manufacturer. Tomosynthesis produces a data set that may be reconstructed in any plane and produces images of inherently higher image contrast than conventional x-ray mammography. This increased image contrast is due to the removal of overlying and underlying tissue utilising the blurring method of tomography.

In breast tomosynthesis (true or false)
- a. A reconstruction technique called filtered back projection may be utilised.
- b. Iterative reconstruction is much more rapid than filtered back projection.
- c. The wide angle of projection increases blurring outside the focal plane.
- d. A truncation image artefact is caused by small breast size.
- e. Breast tissue outside the imaging volume may contribute to the image.

Answers

a. A reconstruction technique called filtered back projection may be utilised.

   True: Filtered back projection is the most commonly used technique in breast tomosynthesis. It is also extensively used in other tomographic specialities.

b. Iterative reconstruction is much more rapid than filtered back projection.

   False: Iterative reconstruction (as its name implies) requires multiple estimations of the calculated final image and for this reason takes longer than the standard filtered back projection technique.

c. The wide angle of projection increases blurring outside the focal plane.

   True: a narrow angle will have the opposite effect.

d. A truncation image artefact is caused by small breast size.

   False: a truncation artefact occurs in magnetic resonance imaging not breast tomosynthesis.

e. Breast tissue outside the imaging volume may contribute to the image.

   True: Overlying and underlying breast tissue, outside the focal plane, may cause reduction in image contrast.

Q2.26 Fluoroscopy

Image quality is a vital concept for diagnostic imaging, but it is more complex than it might appear. For instance, image quality may be poor, but it could be the best that it is possible to achieve and this is often the case in radionuclide imaging. Quality is therefore subjective even though some aspects of the image can be quantified such as spatial or contrast resolution.

When considering, image quality, in fluoroscopy (true or false)
   a. Fluoroscopy is often used as a technique because of its high resolution.
   b. The dose from fluoroscopy can lead to erythema.
   c. In fluoroscopy, contrast is usually as good as digital radiography.
   d. Angiography is a technique for increasing resolution.
   e. Staff dose can be almost eliminated by the use of correct source alignment.

Answers

   a. Fluoroscopy is often used as a technique because of its high resolution.

      False: Although the resolution can be good, it is its dynamic potential that is most useful.

   b. The dose from fluoroscopy can lead to erythema.

      True: Although every effort is made to reduce the skin dose to levels below which erythema is less likely.

   c. In fluoroscopy, contrast is usually as good as digital radiography.

      True: This is especially true where subtraction techniques are used.

   d. Angiography is a technique for increasing resolution.

      False: It increases contrast of blood vessels.

   e. Staff dose can be almost eliminated by the use of correct source alignment.

      False: Dose is still high but it is optimised by the correct source orientation.

Q2.27 Fluoroscopy entrance surface dose

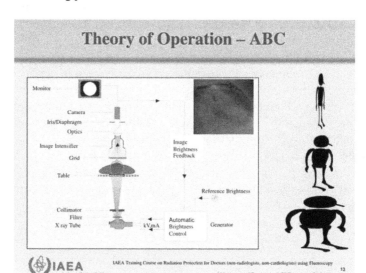

Fluoroscopy, especially interventional, is generally considered to be a high dose technique. There are ways to reduce the dose but the information gained by use of fluoroscopy is so useful that the risk-benefit balance is still in favour of fluoroscopy being used albeit with strict cautions. Attendant staff will also receive doses in excess of those for more conventional plain-film imaging.

In automatic mode fluoroscopy, entrance surface dose (true or false)
   a. When zooming to smaller field size the entrance skin dose usually increases.
   b. Depends on the added filtration.
   c. Is independent of the kV-mA characteristic used.
   d. Doubles if the patient-to-detector distance is halved.
   e. Should not be more than $50\,\mathrm{mGy\,min^{-1}}$ for routine field size.

Answers

a. When zooming to smaller field size the entrance skin dose usually increases.

   True: The entrance dose will vary since the beam intensity is reduced by going to a smaller area but to maintain image quality the system will automatically increase the incident intensity.

b. Depends on the added filtration.

   True: Changing the filtration will affect the beam hardness and hence will affect the photon energies absorbed by the patient.

c. Is independent of the kV-mA characteristic used.

   False: The kV-mA characteristic will alter the beam quality which will in turn change patient dose.

d. Doubles if the patient-to-detector distance is halved.

   False: The distance from source to detector is the important factor in calculations using the inverse square law—in this case this does not alter. In fact, the dose will slightly reduce because of an increase in scatter reaching the detector.

e. Should not be more than $50\,\text{mGy}\,\text{min}^{-1}$ for routine field size.

   True: Although this is a guideline rather than an absolute limit.

IOP Publishing

Scientific Basis of the Royal College of Radiologists Fellowship (2nd Edition)

Illustrated questions and answers

Malcolm Sperrin and John Winder

Chapter 3

Imaging theory

Whilst being aware of the available imaging options, it is also important to be reasonably well versed on basic imaging theory. This relates less to the type of radiation used, to how you describe the processes involved and how you might summarise their performance. This will include factors affecting system resolution, radiation scatter and image contrast and will also require you to have a working knowledge of modulation transfer function as well as a host of other concepts. This is not just abstract. A knowledge of this material enables you have an informed opinion on which modality is most appropriate for given circumstances and is also vital for those whose ambitions extend to imaging research and development.

Q3.1 Digital imaging fundamentals

6	8	6	6	6	110	110	101				
6	7	6	100	120	103	6	7				
6	6	6	100	110	103	6					
5	6	104	110	105	6	7					
6	98	104	107	6	7						
6	103	112	6	6							
101	113	104	6	6							
121	108	6	7								
109	57	5	6								
66	6	6	6								
60	8	8									
7	6	6									

Modern imaging is based upon the representation of human tissue parameters by numbers. These numbers are stored in a matrix and the whole system is known as the digital image. Being based on stored numbers, it is a relatively easy task to manipulate the data to change contrast, edge enhancement, etc, but the size of the discrete regions summarized by the number is also the source of some artefacts such as partial voluming. A basic premise is that the larger the matrix, the smaller the individual element, and hence the image is associated with more detail. The compromise is that the matrix then becomes very large, making storage and manipulation more challenging.

Concerning a digital image matrix (true or false)
a. Individual elements within an image matrix are called pixels.
b. The range of numbers used to represent the image signal is called the dynamic range.
c. The size of an individual pixel is defined by the slice thickness.
d. For a matrix of 256×128 with a square FOV, the pixels will be rectangular.
e. For a fixed FOV, fewer pixels result in greater spatial resolution.

Answers

a. Individual elements within an image matrix are called pixels.

True: The term pixel is derived from 'picture elements'; when considering how an image volume is made up we use the term voxels.

b. The range of numbers used to represent the image signal is called the dynamic range.

True: 8 bit storage (one byte for each pixel value) can store a number between 0–255; 16 bit (2 bytes) can store numbers between 0–65 535.

c. The size of an individual pixel is defined by the slice thickness.

False: An individual pixel size is determined by the image acquisition FOV and the image matrix size. For example a 40×40 cm FOV using a matrix of 512×512 will result in a pixel size of 0.781 mm.

d. For a matrix of 256×128 with a square FOV the pixels will be rectangular.

True: If the square FOV was 256 mm, then the pixel dimensions would be 1.0×2.0 mm.

e. For a fixed FOV, fewer pixels results in greater spatial resolution.

False: Although pixel count is not the only determinant of spatial resolution, we would expect an image to contain more detail and be able to resolve smaller objects with a greater image matrix.

Q3.2 The isotropic voxel

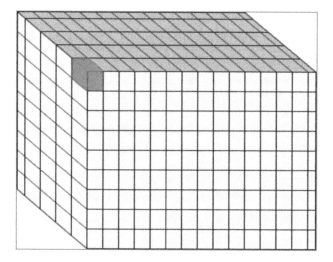

The term isotropy means 'equal in all directions', from the Greek 'isos' which means "equal" and "tropos" which means "way". Therefore, in Radiology, an isotropic voxel is one that has the same dimension in each of the three orthogonal axes. So the following voxel dimension of 0.5 × 05 mm and a 3 mm slice thickness is not isotropic, but one that is 1.0 × 1.0 × 1.0 mm in the x, y, z directions is said to be isotropic. Both CT and MR acquire very nearly isotropic voxels in some image acquisition techniques. Data can easily be interpolated (re-sampled) so that the voxels become isotropic. The advantage of using volumetric data that has isotropic voxels is that image reformats can be created in any of the three orthogonal planes without subsequent loss in image matrix resolution. There may be distinct advantages in using non-isotropic voxels, where the slice thickness is larger than the pixel dimension, as more anatomical coverage will be achieved in the same scan time.

Concerning volumetric data acquisition (true or false)
    a. An isotropic voxel is one where each voxel dimension is different.
    b. A principal benefit of isotropic voxels is that the spatial resolution is equal in each of the orthogonal directions.
    c. A volume containing isotropic voxels must have the same dimensions in the x, y and z directions.
    d. Thinner slices lead to a reduced partial volume artefact.
    e. The stair-step artefact is reduced with isotropic resolution.

Answers

   a. An isotropic voxel is one where each voxel dimension is different.

      False: The definition of isotropic is that 'it has an identical measure of some property in all three dimensions (x, y, z)'. In this case the property is size and a $1.0 \times 1.0 \times 1.0$ mm voxel is said to be isotropic.

   b. A principal benefit of isotropic voxels is that the spatial resolution is equal in each of the orthogonal directions.

      True: Image reformats from axial, sagittal or coronal planes will have the same spatial resolution; images generated from oblique or double oblique planes will have slightly variable resolution due to geometrical considerations.

   c. A volume containing isotropic voxels must have the same dimensions in the x, y and z directions.

      False: A chest–abdomen–pelvis may be $40 \times 40 \times 100$ cm in size but each voxel would be $0.8 \times 0.8 \times 0.8$ mm.

   d. Thinner slices lead to a reduced partial volume artefact.

      True: The partial volume artefact is due to averaging of pixel values within one voxel, if the voxel contains more than one tissue type, then thinner slices have the potential to reduce the number of tissues and reduce the effect of averaging.

   e. The stair-step artefact is reduced with isotropic resolution.

      True: As the slice thickness is reduced for isotropic imaging, the presence of steps between slices (especially in reformats or surface rendering) will be reduced.

Q3.3 Digital image presentation

Digital images are designed to represent detail in a form that makes them suitable for manipulation and analysis by the use of appropriate software. This reduces the size to be displayed such that the eye cannot identify the pixels and also for contrast to be displayed by the use of a grey-scale range.

Concerning digital image presentation (true or false)

    a. There are typically 256 grey levels available for presenting an image on a computer screen.

    b. The eye/brain detector can typically perceive 700–900 individual grey levels in normal room lighting.

    c. A look up table in digital imaging allows the radiologist to measure tissue density.

    d. Digital image noise appears as random fluctuations in pixel values.

    e. A look up table in radiology transforms pixel values into grey levels.

Answers
  a. There are typically 256 grey levels available for presenting an image on a computer screen.
    True: Most computer displays use up to 256 individual grey levels when displaying medical images, although this has increased with the introduction of digital mammographic displays to 1024 grey levels.
  b. They eye/brain detector can typically perceive 700–900 individual grey levels in normal room lighting.
    False: The sensitivity of the eye varies between people and also depends on the background lighting and whether the eye has been dark adapted or not. According to recent research the eye can detect around 720 individual grey levels, but definitely not in normal room conditions. Other image features such as noise and display calibration strongly affect our ability to detect different shades of grey.
  c. A look up table in digital imaging allows the radiologist to measure tissue density.
    False: A look up table is used to relate image pixel values to brightness (or grey level display) on a computer monitor.
  d. Digital image noise appears as random fluctuations in pixel values.
    True: Noise shows up as a speckled or grainy appearance.
  e. A look up table in radiology transforms pixel values into grey levels.
    True: A pixel value or a range of values is assigned a particular grey level as defined by the user during 'windowing' so that the grey levels can be allocated to the appropriate pixel number range to maximize visualization of tissues.

Q3.4 Image digitization

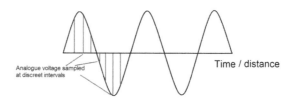

Analogue voltage sampled at discreet intervals

Time / distance

Digitization is the conversion of an analogue voltage (signal measured on a patient) to a number. In imaging the analogue signal is continuously varying and is sampled at discrete intervals. The range from zero signal to the maximum achievable is known as the dynamic range. Depending on the modality this number range may be from 0 to 255, 0 to 65535 and these are known as 8 bit or 16 bit number ranges. These number ranges originate from the storage capacity of computers which is based on the binary numbering system or 1's and 0's. The advantages of digitization are numerous, from storage, transmission, copying of data to processing and manipulation.

The dynamic range of an image (true or false)
    a. Defines the maximum and minimum signals detectable from within the body.
    b. Makes better differentiation between tissues possible when it is smaller.
    c. Can be related to the range of grey levels by a look up table.
    d. Is also called the image depth.
    e. Is generally much greater than the number of grey levels available to represent it on a computer screen.

Answers

a. Defines the maximum and minimum signals detectable from within the body.

True: The dynamic range summarizes the ability of the system either to detect or display the range of grey on the image or the range of intensities being detected. Where the range is very large it may be quoted as a logarithm or as decibels (dB).

b. Makes better differentiation between tissues possible when it is smaller.

False: The extreme case here is that if you only had one grey scale in your dynamic range, then all tissue would appear to be the same. A large dynamic range permits the differences between tissues to be visualized by assigning different grey scale values.

c. Can be related to the range of grey levels by a look up table.

True: A given output parameter may take the form of a voltage, capacitance, etc, and a look up table will assign a portion of the available range to a given grey scale. The more grey scale values that are available the smaller the range of input signal that is assigned and hence there is an increase in the differentiation between tissue types.

d. Is also called the image depth.

True: Depth in this circumstance refers to the number of bits or bytes that are required to store the number range encountered using a particular imaging technique. For instance, CT requires a number range of -1024 to $+3072$ (12 bit storage or two bytes needed for each pixel value).

e. Is generally much greater than the number of grey levels available to represent it on a computer screen.

True: The dynamic range of medical images is increasing all the time and much greater ranges of numbers for signal detection means much greater contrast resolution in an image.

Q3.5 Digital image matrix

The digital image matrix is the framework into which the results of signal digitization are stored. The image matrix is really an array of number s when stored on a workstation. Each element of the image matrix is known as a pixel, derived from picture element. Typical properties of the pixel are its physical dimensions and the dynamic range of pixel values. The image matrix will be defined to have a field of view (FOV) which in MR of the head would be between 220 and 240 mm, whilst in CT, a chest scan will have a field of view of 400 and 500 mm. This means the pixel size in an MR of the head would be 240/256 = 0.9375 mm. The greater the size of the image matrix (512 × 512 has four times the number of pixels as 256 × 256). The dynamic range of each pixel within the image matrix is the range of possible values it can hold. For example, CT numbers typically range from −1024 to +3072, whilst MR may use a number range from 0 to 10 000 or greater.

Concerning digital image matrices (true or false)
  a. The fundamental unit of an image matrix is called a pixel.
  b. The fundamental unit of a three-dimensional volumetric CT scan is called a voxel.
  c. An image with a rectangular FOV must have rectangular pixels.
  d. Pixels with different dimensions along each of the axes are referred to as isotropic.
  e. An isotropic voxel allows the operator to reconstruct images within any orthogonal plane with approximately the same spatial resolution.

Answers
a. The fundamental unit of an image matrix is called a pixel.
   True: The term pixel has been derived from 'picture element'.
b. The fundamental unit of a three-dimensional volumetric CT scan is called a voxel.
   True: The term voxel is derived from 'volume element'.
c. An image with a rectangular FOV must have rectangular pixels.
   False: A rectangular FOV may be filled with square or rectangular pixels and really depends on the modality configuration and imaging parameters.
d. Pixels with different dimensions along each of the axes are referred to as isotropic.
   False: Isotropy defines that the dimensions are the same in any orthogonal direction.
e. An isotropic voxel allows the operator to reconstruct images within any orthogonal plane with approximately the same spatial resolution.
   True: This is approximately true since there may be other factors governing resolution in each of the directions.

Q3.6 Digital image computer displays

The ability to display an image of appropriate quality is crucial to the process of diagnosis. Traditionally film (acetate) was used which had fine grain of silver halide which defined the minimum size of feature that could be visualised within an image. However, film is associated with a 'permanent' image that cannot be altered to allow for exposure errors and furthermore has problems with storage, fire-risk and long-term stability. The use of display screens eliminates the need for film but the limiting factor is now pixel size, dynamic range and brightness to name a few. Ensuring that the display is optimally set up and is also stable with time are vital factors in ensuring a consistent facility on which diagnosis can take place.

Concerning computer digital displays (true or false)
   a. Grey scale monitors typically have better spatial resolution than colour monitors.
   b. A 5 megapixel monitor would use 1024×1280 pixels in its display matrix.
   c. Digital mammography requires the same monitor spatial resolution as MRI.
   d. Displays should be DICOM compliant so that they display patient details.
   e. Pooling is of no significant concern in modern imaging systems.

Answers

a. Grey scale monitors typically have better spatial resolution than colour monitors.

   True: A colour monitor creates the colour effect by the homogenization of three colour emitters which together fool the eye into seeing the required colour. These three emitters will inevitably take up more space than a single emitter just creating a grey scale.

b. A 5 megapixel monitor would use 1024×1280 pixels in its display matrix.

   False: The memory required for the 1024×1024 display is simply 1024^2 which is just over 1 million pixels (megapixels).

c. Digital mammography requires the same monitor spatial resolution as MRI.

   False: Mammography is used to image the finest detail with resolutions down to $20 \, \text{lp mm}^{-1}$. In MRI a typical resolution is $1 \, \text{lp mm}^{-1}$. The mammography system requires monitors with higher resolution.

d. Displays should be DICOM compliant so that they display patient details.

   False: In this case DICOM compliance refers to the grey scale calibration of the monitor so that image display is consistent across an organization.

e. Pooling is of no significant concern in modern imaging systems.

   True: Pooling refers to the limited display of one grey level where more data are available but the monitor cannot present a range of shades of grey. In modern systems, pooling is theoretically possible, but the default settings will avoid pooling.

Q3.7 Spatial resolution in imaging systems

10 lp cm^{-1} 5 lp cm^{-1} 3 lp cm^{-1} 2 lp cm^{-1} 1 lp cm^{-1}

The ability of an imaging system to detect and display small details (and sharp edges) is termed its spatial resolution. The spatial resolution is dependent on many factors, the modality and image matrix dimensions are only one part of the chain. We use pairs of signals (signal/no signal or black/white or dense/not dense) detectable by the system at varying sizes and we define this as line pairs per distance (lp cm^{-1} or lp mm^{-1}).

What are the typical spatial resolutions for the following imaging systems?
    a. CT.
    b. MR.
    c. Digital mammography.
    d. CR.
    e. PET.

Answers

a. CT: 6–20 lp cm^{-1}.

This value depends on the image matrix, the reconstruction algorithm and the detector spacing. Typically, for a scan with a 40 cm FOV and a 512 × 512 matrix, the pixel size is 0.8 mm, which relates to a spatial resolution of 6 lp cm^{-1}.

b. MR: 5–7 lp cm^{-1}.

MR is a lower resolution modality than people think, its image quality is due to high inherent soft tissue contrast.

c. Digital mammography: 20 lp mm^{-1}.

One of the main purposes of mammography is to detect very small deposits of calcification which may indicate the presence of a tumour and therefore a very high spatial resolution is required.

d. CR: 3–6 lp cm^{-1}.

This depends on the imaging plate size but will range from 3–6 lp cm^{-1}, the former for small plates and the latter for larger plates.

e. PET: 1 lp cm^{-1}.

The spatial resolution of nuclear medicine systems is low compared to other imaging modalities.

Q3.8 Picture archive and communication system I

The storage and transmission of digital medical images has had a profound effect on data management within radiology. The major components of a picture archive and communication system (PACS) are as follows: the IT networks for transport of image and patient data; the image database and image processing; the short- and long-term storage systems and the display systems. International standards have been established which define important aspects of digital image transmission, manipulation, display and storage to enable the sharing of all radiological images throughout the healthcare system.

In a picture archive and communication system (true or false)
  a. Display monitors should be quality assured to ensure consistent image quality.
  b. Medical images requiring fast access should be stored on a long-term archive.
  c. The text data storage is much larger than the image data storage.
  d. The DICOM standard governs the transfer of patient notes around the hospital.
  e. HL7 standard defines the transmission of MR images to wards.

Answers

a. Display monitors should be quality assured to ensure consistent image quality.

True: To ensure that medical images look similar across a healthcare institution (ambient lighting conditions will vary from one place to another) display monitors should be regularly tested and calibrated for brightness, contrast and spatial resolution. This also ensures that the monitors present the necessary information consistent with the modality of choice.

b. Medical images requiring fast access should be stored on a long-term archive.

False: The long-term archive in a PACS may be magnetic tape or disk based and be routinely off-line, therefore images that are required to be accessed quickly should be stored on hard disk or flash media.

c. The text data storage is much larger than the image data storage.

False: Text storage may require thousands of bytes (kB), whereas medical images may require millions of bytes (megabytes, MB) or billions of bytes (gigabytes, GB).

d. The DICOM standard governs the transfer of patient notes around the hospital.

False: The DICOM standard is used for the transfer of medical images, not patient notes, around the hospital. Electronic patient records is a second IT system with complex architecture and protocols.

e. HL7 standard defines the transmission of MR images to wards.

False: HL7 defines how text information is transferred around the hospital network.

Q3.9 Picture archive and communication system II

Image display workstations are categorised by their modality image review and quality assurance, in diagnostic reporting, and display at a clinical level for review purposes. Diagnostic reporting workstations are of the highest quality in terms of image display (resolution and brightness) and image manipulation functions. Monitors for reviewing images at a clinical level require lower quality systems where images may be reviewed within web browsing technology on standard desktop computers. Quality assurance of medical image display monitors ensures that digital images are presented to the same standard across the clinical environment (ambient display and lighting conditions are relevant).

Regarding performance of picture archive and communication system monitors (true or false)

   a. A two-megapixel monitor would be suitable to display digital mammographic images.
   b. A one-megapixel monitor will display four CT scans simultaneously.
   c. Screen contrast is effectively improved in a darkened viewing room.
   d. Pixel pitch refers to the overall screen dimensions.
   e. A DICOM calibrated screen has a luminance of 500–600 cd m^{-2}.

Answers

    a. A two-megapixel monitor would be suitable to display digital mammo-graphic images.

        False: A digital mammographic image is typically 6000 × 4500 pixels, which would normally be displayed on a five-megapixel monitor and this limitation is such that this would not display the full image. The required pixel density can be calculated as follows: the resolution required is 10 lp mm^{-1} or better or a pixel size of 0.05 mm. If the monitor is 50 cm × 70 cm this leads to 5000 × 7000 pixels.

    b. A one-megapixel monitor will display four CT scans simultaneously.

        True: A one-megapixel monitor is typically 1280 × 1024 pixels. A CT image is 512 × 512 pixels, therefore four CT images could be fully displayed.

    c. Screen contrast is effectively improved in a darkened viewing room.

        True: In a well-lit room the dark state of the display is not as dark as when it is viewed in an unlit room, therefore reduction in contrast is experienced due to ambient light.

    d. Pixel pitch refers to the overall screen dimensions.

        False: Pixel pitch refers to the number of pixels over a given distance or the pixel density.

    e. A DICOM calibrated screen has a luminance of 500–600 cd m^{-2}.

        True: Display monitors range from around 100 cd m^{-2} to ultra-bright monitors that can be viewed in direct sunlight at 2500 cd m^{-2}.

Q3.10 Image quality

Noise = 3.0
(Standard
Deviation)

Noise = 10.0
(Standard
Deviation)

Image quality is defined by three basic measures. Image noise: measured as the standard deviation of pixel values within a defined region in an image. Image contrast: the difference in signal strength between two adjacent regions within an image. Spatial resolution: the ability to resolve small objects or edges within an image. These quantities are very variable between medical imaging modalities and vary within an individual image. Therefore, there may be high contrast within one part of the image and low contrast within another part of the image. It is preferable to have high contrast between disease and normal tissue to increase visibility.

Concerning image quality (true or false)
   a. Images with a high signal-to-noise ratio demonstrate small objects more clearly.
   b. Image low signal-to-noise ratio is an indication of poorer image quality.
   c. Signal averaging increases image signal to noise.
   d. As image contrast decreases the image contains more black and white grey levels.
   e. In medical imaging it is preferable to have a low contrast-to-noise ratio.

Answers

a. Images with a high signal-to-noise ratio demonstrate small objects more clearly.

   True: The higher the signal-to-noise ratio the better the image quality and therefore details will be better visualised.

b. Image low signal-to-noise ratio is an indication of poorer image quality.

   True: Lower signal to noise means a proportionately greater amount of noise or graininess, which is undesirable.

c. Signal averaging increases image signal to noise.

   True: Signal averaging results in reduced noise as it is a random signal and partially cancels itself out.

d. As image contrast decreases the image becomes more black and white.

   False: Greater black and white content produces the appearance of higher image contrast.

e. In medical imaging it is preferable to have a low contrast-to-noise ratio.

   False: A high contrast-to-noise ratio is preferable in medical imaging as it increases contrast between disease and normal tissue and low noise produces better image quality.

Q3.11 Partial volume effect

Object in
image matrix

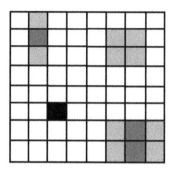

Pixel grey scale
due to partial
volume effect

The partial volume effect occurs in both 2D and 3D imaging systems. When a pixel or voxel is only partially filled with signal from one tissue type (for example, bone), then the resultant image suffers from reduced contrast when representing the tissue. The pixel value is calculated from the contributions of two or more tissues that exist within the pixel. The partial volume effect may result in loss of image contrast, loss of edge sharpness (or blurring) or apparent reduced activity in radionuclide studies.

The partial volume effect (true or false)
  a. Decreases image contrast.
  b. Decreases with increased slice acquisition thickness.
  c. Causes image edges within images to become blurred.
  d. In MRI, can be reduced by changing the slice thickness from 4 mm to 2 mm.
  e. Is defined by the detector configuration in CT scanning.

Answers
a. Decreases image contrast.
    True: The signal from a small high contrast object will be smeared over a number of pixels, therefore contrast will be reduced (see diagram).
b. Decreases with increased slice acquisition thickness.
    False: The partial volume effect will increase with increased slice thickness.
c. Causes image edges within images to become blurred.
    True: See diagram above where a small object becomes blurred due to the partial volume effect. The objects borders become less sharp.
d. In MRI, can be reduced by changing the slice thickness from 4 mm to 2 mm.
    True: A thinner slice thickness reduces the partial volume effect.
e. Is defined by the detector configuration in CT scanning.
    True: In a multi-slice CT detector the individual detector elements impact on the partial volume effect.

Q3.12 Image processing in radiological imaging

Image processing occurs during all aspects of image data acquisition to image display. During the acquisition of CT image raw data, a digital mathematical filter is applied to reduce artefacts and enhance image quality. Simple processing steps like adding images together or subtracting images pre- and post-addition of contrast media are used after data acquisition. Edge enhancement may be applied for image display to increase image contrast of edges, especially for bone. The adjustment of image contrast and brightness using image windowing is routinely applied during the display process.

Concerning image processing in radiology (true or false)
  a. Image addition is used to increase image noise.
  b. Image subtraction increases image contrast.
  c. Image registration may produce tissue edge artefacts.
  d. Image edge enhancement increases image noise.
  e. Image compression can result in changes to image detail.

Answers
   a. Image addition is used to increase image noise.
      False: Image addition is the same as signal averaging and therefore reduces image noise.
   b. Image subtraction increases image contrast.
      True: Image subtraction is routinely used in digital subtraction angiography and produces an increase in blood vessel contrast.
   c. Image registration may produce tissue edge artefacts.
      True: Image registration is the mapping together of two images of the same anatomical location (from the same or different modalities). However, if the registration is not accurate or the images are distorted edge artefacts may occur.
   d. Image edge enhancement increases image noise.
      True: Most, if not all, image edge enhancement processes will increase image noise whilst sharpening edges.
   e. Image compression can result in changes to image detail.
      True: In lossless compression no image detail is changed, however, where a 'lossy' compression technique is used, image detail may be discarded by the mathematical process.

Q3.13 Spatial resolution in medical imaging

Spatial resolution test object

In radiology, spatial resolution refers to the ability of an imaging system to differentiate in two high contrast objects. In terms of an imaging system, we are referring to the initial detection of the signal, conversion of the signal into a different energy form (for example, gamma rays to light photons), data filtering and processing and the final image display device. Each system stage may impact on the overall modality resolution. If two objects are not clearly resolved, then they will appear as one object.

Regarding spatial resolution in medical imaging (true or false)
   a. Pixel size and spatial resolution measure the same aspect of image quality.
   b. CT is a generally lower spatial resolution modality compared to MRI.
   c. Fluoroscopic imaging has a lower spatial resolution than digital mammography.
   d. Spatial resolution can be measured in line pairs per millimetre (lp mm^{-1}) across all modalities.
   e. X-ray tube focal spot size can impact on spatial resolution.

Answers

a. Pixel size and spatial resolution measure the same aspect of image quality.

False: Pixel size may impact on spatial resolution but there are generally other system properties that also impact on spatial resolution, for example data sampling, slice thickness and detector size.

b. CT is a generally lower spatial resolution modality compared to MRI.

False: Computed tomography will generally have better spatial resolution than magnetic resonance imaging although the latter is improving all the time (5 lp mm^{-1} compared to 2 lp mm^{-1}).

c. Fluoroscopic imaging has a lower spatial resolution than digital mammography.

True: Digital mammography has a spatial resolution of 20 lp mm^{-1}, whereas, fluoroscopy produces about 2 lp mm^{-1} resolution.

d. Spatial resolution can be measured in lp mm^{-1} across all modalities.

True: Line pairs per millimetre is the standard measurement of spatial resolution across all imaging systems.

e. X-ray tube focal spot size can impact on spatial resolution.

True: A small focal spot size will result in improved spatial resolution.

Q3.14 Multimodality imaging

Multi-modality imaging describes the combination of information from a range of different imaging techniques. The information may be in the form of anatomy, physiology or physical property. The image data may be acquired sequentially, using separate imaging devices, usually at different times. The images from these two systems are then combined or fused together using specialist software and mathematical techniques such as image registration. Another methodology uses an imaging device where two separate modalities are combined into one system and images are acquired during the same examination. In this case the images are acquired close together in time and the patient remains in the same position on the same couch.

Regarding multimodality imaging (true or false)
- a. Patient image data may be acquired sequentially from different modalities and 'fused' using software.
- b. The two modalities being fused must be of the same resolution.
- c. Images must be acquired from the same modality on different days.
- d. Functional and anatomical data are combined to produce a hybrid image.
- e. Image alignment is a fundamental step in the process.

Answers

a. Patient image data may be acquired sequentially from different modalities and 'fused' using software.
> **True:** Images may be acquired minutes or hours apart and spatially registered using specialist software.

b. The two modalities being fused must be of the same resolution.
> **False:** The modalities can have very different resolution, as with PET and CT, as the lower resolution modality may be subsampled to match the other data set.

c. Images must be acquired from the same modality on different days.
> **False:** Images may be acquired from different modalities, days apart, or from the same modality.

d. Functional and anatomical data are combined to produce a hybrid image.
> **True:** Examples of this are PET and CT or SPECT and CT, where the functional activity of one modality is placed within the anatomy of CT.

e. Image alignment is a fundamental step in the process.
> **True:** Image alignment, also known as image registration, is a fundamental step where rotation, translation, scaling and correction for image distortion may be employed.

Q3.15 Common imaging themes I

It is very common to enlarge or magnify an image. This may arise for one of a number of reasons and can be achieved by the use of a hand magnifier but generally available software or by the use of options embedded within a PACS system. There is a fundamental difference between magnifying a section of an image from a previously stored original as opposed to magnifying the displayed image prior to storage. The difference is analogous to domestic circumstances where a large lens can be used on a camera to magnify a scene as opposed to using a small lens and then using a magnifying glass on the printed image. Understanding the benefits and detriments of these options is an important aspect of optimising the diagnostic value of the contents of the image.

Considering the effects of magnification (true or false)
    a. Magnification of a stored image reveals detail that was previously unrecorded.
    b. An MTF with a high cut-off frequency implies a high magnification.
    c. The highest resolution in an image that has been magnified from a live image source will be degraded if the image is frozen.
    d. The resolution contained within an image can be enhanced by post-processing.
    e. Contrast and magnification are inversely related.

Answers

a. Magnification of a stored image reveals detail that was previously unrecorded.

  False: If the image is stored then magnifying it can only increase the size of what is already there. It will already have been recorded and whilst it might be more apparent, it is not new information.

b. An MTF with a high cut-off frequency implies a high magnification.

  False: The MTF cut-off frequency is independent of magnification. This confusion sometimes arises because in some images, magnification can reveal small detail, but it is information that is already present and is not created or modified by magnification.

c. The highest resolution in an image that has been magnified from a live image source will be degraded if the image is frozen.

  False: Freezing the image will simply store what is being viewed. However, if the image is stored, especially using image compression, then the image can be degraded.

d. The resolution contained within an image can be enhanced by post-processing.

  False: Post processing will select those features in the image that are more useful and at best they leave the basic image features unchanged. It is more common for post-processing to degrade the image even if only in a subtle way.

e. Contrast and magnification are inversely related.

  False: Contrast and resolution are independent. Some confusion arises because features can become more visible when the contrast is increased but the relationship is more complex than one simply being the inverse of the other.

Q3.16 Common imaging themes II

Spatial resolution in an image is one of the primary considerations relating to how the image can be used for diagnostic purposes There are many factors that contribute to the final spatial resolution of an image such as detector performance, movement and reconstruction methods. Furthermore, there are many factors that affect the ability of the observer to identify such features and hence standardised techniques exist to assess the best resolution in the image.

With reference to spatial resolution (true or false)
a. Increasing the spatial density of detectors generally improves resolution in the final image.
b. Spatial resolution can be improved by increasing the contrast.
c. The modulation transfer function (MTF) can be used to derive the limiting resolution in an image.
d. PET and CT modalities are often hybridised because their resolutions are comparable.
e. The spatial resolution in an image can be calculated by use of a sharp, high-contrast edge.

Answers

a. Increasing the spatial density of detectors generally improves resolution in the final image.

True: Not always, but generally. The important point here is that the limiting factor on imaging system resolution is the design of the equipment. This is not the case with ultrasound where the limiting resolution is usually taken to be a multiple of the wavelength.

b. Spatial resolution can be improved by increasing the contrast.

False: Contrast and spatial resolution are largely independent although if the contrast is increased, some features can be easier to see.

c. The modulation transfer function (MTF) can be used to derive the limiting resolution in an image.

True: The MTF curve crosses the horizontal (y) axis at the highest spatial resolution. This may not be easily visible in the image due to the limiting resolution being associated with features of low modulation.

d. PET and CT modalities are often hybridised because their resolutions are comparable.

False: Their resolutions are very different. They are usually selected so as for one to be functional and the other to be anatomical.

e. The spatial resolution in an image can be calculated by use of a sharp, high-contrast edge.

True: This is a standard technique.

Q3.17 Common imaging themes III

Any image can contain information that is not possible to separate out from all of the other information surrounding it. Furthermore, the presence of some forms of detail can be a distraction from the information that is of most use to the clinician. Image processing enables some aspects of the image to be removed or enhanced according to need. This could simply be the removal of certain colours as you would with a filter but there are many other more involved techniques that permit the selective enhancement of features of interest, whether they be edges or bone structures, for instance. Image processing is applied during or after the image acquisition stage and when it occurs is of importance to the on-going intentions of the image.

When using image processing (true or false)
    a. It is important to process stored images rather than the original in order to revert back to the original should the processing be ineffective.
    b. Processing an image generates truly new data.
    c. The use of gamma curves is one example of image processing.
    d. Processing images can lead to the loss of detail.
    e. Doppler imaging is a processing technique.

Answers

   a. It is important to process stored images rather than the original in order to revert back to the original should the processing be ineffective.

      True: if you modify the live image and then store it, you cannot revert back to the original data without taking the image again.

   b. Processing an image generates truly new data.

      False: the processed image will be based on what data in the original image you select to display, hence it is not really new data.

   c. The use of gamma curves is one example of image processing.

      True: The gamma curve assigns a grey scale to the signal from the detector output. You can select the form of the gamma curve.

   d. Processing images can lead to the loss of detail.

      True: Consider, for instance, edge enhancement. You are selecting the edge and reducing the rest of the data that is less important to you.

   e. Doppler imaging is a processing technique.

      True: This is not really about how the Doppler signal is calculated but rather the fact that it is used to overlay the image as a colour flow map.

Q3.18 Modulation transfer function

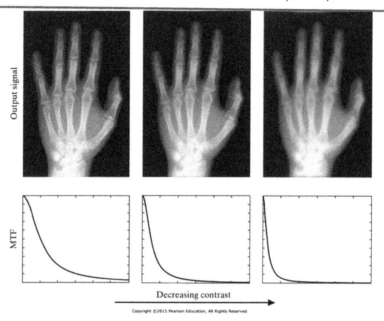

Most users of imaging systems will have seen images that appear to be substandard either in comparison to other scanners or perhaps the quality appears to be dropping with time. Such subjective assessment, whilst of some use, is difficult to use to more precisely to identify a change in performance because it is non-specific and subject to many influences additional to the system's intrinsic performance. One method that does permit more objective analysis is to analyse the spatial frequencies in the image and see how they change between systems and over time.

Considering the Modulation Transfer Function (MTF) (true or false)

    a. The modulation transfer function (MTF) by default has a value of 1 for 0 lp mm^{-1}.

    b. The area under the MTF curve provides important information about total energy dissipated.

    c. A typical MTF for breast imaging would contain higher spatial frequencies than that observed for general x-ray imaging.

    d. The concept of MTF cannot apply to the human eye because of accommodation by the lens.

    e. In MRI, T1 and T2 images would be expected to have different MTF profiles.

Answers

   a. The modulation transfer function (MTF) by default has a value of 1 for 0 lp mm^{-1}.

      True: This can be seen in the simplest terms as just the difference between peak black and peak white.

   b. The area under the MTF curve provides important information about total energy dissipated.

      False: The area under the MTF curve has no practical meaning. It is the curve shape that is relevant.

   c. A typical MTF for breast imaging would contain higher spatial frequencies than that observed for general x-ray imaging.

      True: Mammography sets have a fine focal point which leads to the higher resolution necessary for imaging small detail. This equates to a higher spatial frequency and hence the cut off is further to the right on the spatial frequency (Y) axis.

   d. The concept of MTF cannot apply to the human eye because of accommodation by the lens.

      False: MTF can be used for any imaging system. It is simply a graphical visualisation of the detail that can be seen and applies equally to the eye as to other imaging systems.

   e. In MRI, T1 and T2 images would be expected to have different MTF profiles.

      False: The spatial frequency in an MRI image is defined by the gradients, RF pulse design, image matrix and not the type of pulse sequence used.

IOP Publishing

Scientific Basis of the Royal College of Radiologists Fellowship (2nd Edition)

Illustrated questions and answers

Malcolm Sperrin and John Winder

Chapter 4

Radiation protection

Whilst using ionizing radiation for imaging it is not sufficient to obtain a high quality image. It is important to obtain an image that is diagnostically useful and for purpose. There is well-established risks associated with the use of ionizing radiation and much effort is conducted to minimise the risks to patient and staff alike. This risk-benefit analysis for use of ioising radiation is complex and it is vital for you to have a comprehensive working knowledge of the key issues since you need to ensure that the

doi:10.1088/978-0-7503-2148-8ch4

patient receives benefit from the imaging modality that you prescribe. There is potential to open up the prospect of litigation from one or more different Acts some of which are generic and some relate specifically to medical exposure. Some of this drive for tight control arises because there is no possibility of removing the health detriment from radiation exposure and furthermore the effect is broadly considered to be cumulative.

Q4.1 Radiation dose reduction in pregnancy

The risk to the foetus due to exposure to radiation during medical examinations is generally low for routine x-rays of the hips, abdomen and lower back, however, other examinations like CT scans or nuclear medicine scans may increase the risk due to the higher dose of radiation used. The foetus is regarded as a member of the public and therefore the exposure limit for the foetus of a pregnant member of staff is 1 mSv per annum which is the same as that for a member of the public. There is a further dose limit to the abdomen of the pregnant member of staff of 13 mSv over a three month period to ensure that any potential dose received is not concentrated over a short period of time.

Concerning a pregnant member of staff (true or false)
    a. The foetus should never be exposed to ionizing radiation.
    b. The limit of exposure to the abdomen of a female employee of reproductive capacity is 30 mSv annually.
    c. The woman should stop operating ionizing radiation based equipment as soon as they know they are pregnant.
    d. The woman should inform her employer within three months of knowing she is pregnant.
    e. Certain types of staff are at higher risk of radiation exposure during pregnancy than others.

Answers

a. The foetus should never be exposed to ionizing radiation.

   False: It is required that the foetus should not be exposed to any significant risk through ionizing radiation. To this end, a dose limit to the foetus is set to that of a member of the public (annual dose limit of 1 mSv) and is applied over the relevant declared pregnancy term, that is, from the point in time that the employee tells their employer about the pregnancy.

b. The limit of exposure to the abdomen of a female employee of reproductive capacity is 30 mSv annually.

   False: The limit is 13 mSv over any consecutive 3 month period.

c. They should stop operating ionizing radiation based equipment as soon as they know they are pregnant.

   False: As the limit for foetal exposure during pregnancy is set at 1 mSv, it is highly unlikely that they would be exposed to such an amount of radiation.

d. The woman should inform her employer within three months of knowing she is pregnant.

   False: The woman should inform her employer in writing as soon as she her pregnancy is confirmed.

e. Certain types of staff are at higher risk of radiation exposure during pregnancy than others.

   True: Evidence shows that interventional radiologists and cardiologists receive a higher average radiation dose than the majority of other staff working with diagnostic x-rays. Vascular surgeons are also likely to be exposed to higher amounts of radiation.

Q4.2 The ALARA principle

The International Commission on Radiological Protection (ICRP, www.icrp.org) is an international independent organization which provides recommendations and guidance on all aspects of radiation protection (not just medical). The key principles that have been adopted are as follows: no practice should be adopted unless it produces a net benefit to the patient, all exposures should be as low as reasonably achievable (ALARA) and doses to individuals should not exceed limits. There is a responsibility on healthcare institutions to abide by the Ionizing Radiations Regulations (IRR; 1999) and the Ionizing Radiation (Medical Exposure) Regulations (IRMER; 2000). An employer is responsible for designation of controlled areas, and should consult with a radiation protection adviser on adherence to the regulations and quality assurance (QA) of equipment.

Concerning the ALARA principle (true or false)
   a. ALARA requires that all radiation exposures should be as low as possible.
   b. Every patient must have gonad, eye, breast and thyroid protection during a CT scan.
   c. Staff should stop operating ionizing radiation based equipment as soon as they know they are pregnant.
   d. The woman should inform her employer within three months of knowing she is pregnant.
   e. Certain types of staff are at higher risk of radiation exposure during pregnancy than others.

Answers

a. ALARA requires that all radiation exposures should be as low as possible.

False: The principle 'As Low As Reasonably Achievable' is in the context of taking into account economic and social factors, so it is not an outright principle. This also means that there are no radiation exposure limits for patients.

b. Every patient must have gonad, eye, breast, and thyroid protection during a CT scan.

False: It would be ideal for full protection to be afforded to every patient, however, economic limitations may mean that this is not always possible.

c. Staff should stop operating ionizing radiation based equipment as soon as they know they are pregnant.

False: The limit for foetal exposure during pregnancy is set at 1 mSv and it is highly unlikely that they would be exposed to such an amount of radiation in the working environment.

d. The woman should inform her employer within three months of knowing she is pregnant.

False: the woman should inform her employer in writing as soon as her pregnancy is confirmed.

e. Certain types of staff are at higher risk of radiation exposure during pregnancy than others.

True: Evidence shows that interventional radiologists and cardiologists receive higher average radiation dose than the majority of other staff working with diagnostic x-rays. Vascular surgeons are also likely to be exposed to higher amounts of radiation.

Q4.3 Types of radiation effects

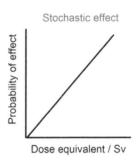

We categorize the effects of radiation into two different effects: deterministic and stochastic. Deterministic means there is a threshold of radiation dose below which the effect does not occur, however, once the threshold dose is passed the severity of the effect increases very rapidly. For example, skin erythema, ulceration, hair loss, sterility and cataracts are all examples of deterministic effects. Some effects, like the formation of cataracts, are cumulative, therefore it is important to monitor eye exposure over a subject's lifetime (when having multiple CT scans of the head). Stochastic effects are those where the effect happens by chance and the probability that the effect will occur increases linearly with radiation dose. It is generally accepted that the risk of the effect occurring (development of cancer for example) is there even at very small doses, however, the severity of the effect does not change.

Concerning deterministic effects (true or false)
a. The threshold for a deterministic (non-stochastic) effect varies between individuals.
b. Deterministic effects may be cumulative.
c. The majority of deterministic effects occur above 10 grays (Gy).
d. It is highly unlikely that deterministic effects will occur at the radiation doses found in diagnostic radiology.
e. Deterministic effects do not affect the foetus.

Answers

a. The threshold for a deterministic (non-stochastic) effect varies between individuals.

   True: Their effects are characterized as having a threshold radiation dose below which the effect does not occur, however, once the threshold is met or exceeded the probability of it occurring increases very rapidly to a level where it will more than likely occur.

b. Deterministic effects may be cumulative.

   True: The formation of a cataract (deterministic effect) in the eye occurs above a threshold of approximately 5 Gy and the effect is cumulative. Therefore another exposure of 5 Gy at another time will result in greater or more cataract formation. People working in areas of high radiation exposure should be monitored carefully over their lifetime.

c. The majority of deterministic effects occur above 10 Gy.

   False: Deterministic effects such as skin erythema (2–5 Gy), hair loss (2–5 Gy) and sterility (2–3 Gy) all occur well below 10 Gy. This value is an absorbed dose and does not take into account the radiation type or the organ sensitivity which would be measured in sieverts.

d. It is highly unlikely that deterministic effects will occur at the radiation doses found in diagnostic radiology.

   False: For general diagnostic examinations absorbed doses range from 0.1 mGy to 50 mGy depending on the modality and range of the anatomy imaged, which is well below the threshold for deterministic effects. However, some complex interventional radiology examinations use high skin doses of up to 50 mGy per minute and last over an hour, therefore resulting in doses in excess of a deterministic threshold (3 Gy in this case). It is not unheard of for patients to receive skin burns and hair loss through interventional procedures.

e. Deterministic effects do not affect the foetus.

   False: The threshold for deterministic effects on the foetus is between 100–500 mGy (much lower that observed in the adult).

Q4.4 Stochastic effects of radiation

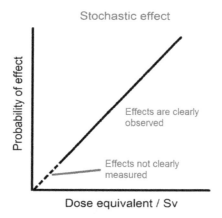

The variation of risk as a function of exposure is complex and open to debate. However, data from bomb survivors and those having undergone other forms of radiation exposure leads to current best practice.

Concerning stochastic effects (true or false)
    a. A stochastic effect is one that will definitely occur.
    b. The two main stochastic effects are carcinogenesis and genetic abnormalities.
    c. Radiation exposed tissue risk factors are constant.
    d. It is highly unlikely that stochastic effects will occur at the radiation doses found in diagnostic radiology.
    e. The stochastic risk for children is twice that of adults.

Answers

a. A stochastic effect is one that will definitely occur.

False: The term stochastic means that the effect will happen by chance and there is a recognized probability that it will occur. The severity of the effect does not increase with a greater amount of radiation, just the probability of it occurring.

b. The two main stochastic effects are carcinogenesis and genetic abnormalities.

True: It has been clearly demonstrated (from historical studies of large radiation incidents) that there is a greater number of cancers in a population of people exposed to higher radiation doses than the unexposed population. The genetic risk is more difficult to assess and the evidence less convincing. Children of parents who were exposed to large radiation doses have not (as yet) been demonstrated to have a higher incidence of genetic abnormality than the rest of the population.

c. Radiation exposed tissue risk factors are constant.

False: Risk factors for body tissues take into account the risk of death (not just that of contracting cancer) and vary throughout the body. They typically range from 0.01 for skin to 0.2 for gonads. This means that if the skin is exposed to the same dose as the gonads, the probability is 20 times greater that an effect on the gonads will occur compared to the skin.

d. It is highly unlikely that stochastic effects will occur at the radiation doses found in diagnostic radiology.

False: This depends on what you mean by highly unlikely. Typically, if there is the predicted linear relationship between dose and probability of death by cancer, then for a population of 20 000 people exposed to a whole body dose of 1 mSv (diagnostic dose), there will be one excess death due to cancer. Over the population of a large country this could amount to hundreds of people.

e. The stochastic risk for children is twice that of adults.

False: Data from mothers who had x-rays of the abdomen during pregnancy indicate that an exposed foetus/child is between eight and ten times more at risk that an adult.

Q4.5 Absorbed dose

It is important to know the total radiation delivered to a patient for all types of medical imaging examinations. The unit is absorbed dose and measured in grays, which is joules per kilogram. However, this parameter does not take into account the effect of different types of radiation (radiobiological effectiveness) and also the radiosensitivity of different tissues (effective dose). The impact of different types of radiation is accounted for by introducing a weighting factor, known as the *quality factor*, which is used to generate the equivalent dose.

Concerning ionizing radiation (true or false)
   a. Alpha particles have a quality factor of around 20 compared to x-rays.
   b. The greater the quality factor the greater the relative impact of the radiation, i.e. the damage that it may cause.
   c. One gray is the absorption of one joule of energy per one kilogram of tissue.
   d. The sievert is the amount of energy deposited per unit kilogram (J kg^{-1}) and adjusted by a weighting factor.
   e. Weighting factors in radiation protection are used for radiation type and amount of radiation.

Answers

    a. Alpha particles have a quality factor of around 20 compared to x-rays.

        True: The quality factor for x-rays is 1, therefore the effect of alpha particles is 20 times greater than that of x-rays.

    b. The greater the quality factor the greater the relative impact of the radiation, i.e. the damage that it may cause.

        True: As the quality factor becomes greater so does the amount of energy that it deposits within the tissue.

    c. One gray is the absorption of one joule of energy per one kilogram of tissue.

        True: The unit for grays is $J\ kg^{-1}$.

    d. The sievert is the amount of energy deposited per unit kilogram ($J\ kg^{-1}$).

        True: This is the same unit as used for grays, however, it is affected by the tissue weighting factor and also any other dose modifying factors like dose rate, fractionation and the non-uniform distribution of dose throughout a tissue volume.

    e. Weighting factors in radiation protection are used for radiation type and amount of radiation.

        False: Weighting factors in radiological protection (W_R and W_T) are for types of radiation and for types of tissue.

Q4.6 Dose area product

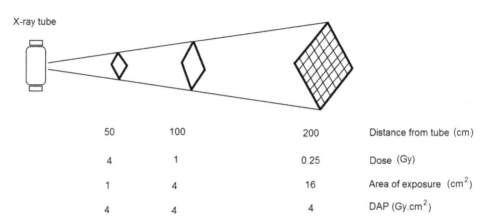

	50	100		200	Distance from tube (cm)
	4	1		0.25	Dose (Gy)
	1	4		16	Area of exposure (cm^2)
	4	4		4	DAP (Gy.cm^2)

A dose area product (DAP) meter is a useful device for measuring dose to the patient. It consists of an ionization chamber and some electronics to capture the radiation dose. The output is the radiation dose to air (air kerma) times the area of the x-ray field. It is a useful device for measuring dose due to single exposures or can be used for more complex examinations like fluoroscopy or multiple radiographs where the total dose is integrated over the procedure. The figure shows how DAP is independent of the distance of the subject from the source of the x-rays, as it is the product of the dose and the area of the exposure.

DAP (true or false)
a. Is proportional to the square of the distance from the focus of the x-ray tube.
b. Can be measured using an ionization chamber attached to the exit port of the x-ray tube.
c. Generates a measure of dose with units of Gy cm^{-2}.
d. Produces an appropriate quantity for dosimetry in fluoroscopy.
e. May be used to set diagnostic reference levels.

Answers

a. Is proportional to the square of the distance from the focus of the x-ray tube.

   False: DAP does not depend on the distance from the x-ray focus to the subject.

b. Can be measured using an ionization chamber attached to the exit port of the x-ray tube.

   True: A DAP is normally positioned after the exit window of the x-ray tube where it will capture all the x-rays. It also takes into account the anode heel effect and any added filtration which would normally be added to the x-ray beam before the DAP meter.

c. Generates a measure of dose with units of $Gy\ cm^{-2}$.

   False: The unit is $Gy\ cm^2$ as the minus sign would indicate that the measurement is dose per unit area but is actually dose times unit area.

d. Produces an appropriate quantity for dosimetry in fluoroscopy.

   True: The DAP meter can measure accumulated x-ray exposure for individual exposures and also for fluoroscopy, producing a final figure that is the integral of all exposures.

e. May be used to set diagnostic reference levels.

   True: ICRP recommend that readings from DAP meters providing dose measurement in $mGy\ cm^2$ should be used to establish diagnostic reference levels to improve regional and national doses for x-ray examinations.

Q4.7 Radiation controlled areas

**RADIATION
SUPERVISED AREA**

RISK OF RADIATION

The designation of physical areas is an important part of radiation protection. A controlled area is one where staff need to follow specific or special procedures which restrict exposure or prevent or limit the chance of a radiation accident, or where the exposure is likely to exceed 6 mSv per annum or at least three tenths of any relevant radiation dose limit. Examples of controlled areas are x-ray rooms and areas where radionuclides are administered. A supervised area is one that requires continual monitoring to determine the area's status with regard to designation or where a person is likely to receive an effective dose greater than 1 mSv per annum or a dose greater than one tenth of any relevant dose limit.

Concerning controlled and supervised areas (true or false)
  a. Only a classified person may enter a controlled area.
  b. Controlled and supervised areas should be identified in the local rules.
  c. The radiation protection supervisor (RPS) is responsible for staff complying with local rules.
  d. Controlled and supervised areas should have a warning sign and indicate the nature of the hazard above the door.
  e. Controlled and supervised areas are not required for mobile examinations.

Answers

    a. Only a classified person may enter a controlled area.

        False: Classified workers (those who are likely to be exposed to greater than three tenths of exposure limits) can enter a controlled area, but workers for other employers, such as engineers or service personnel, can also enter in accordance with local written protocols.

    b. Controlled and supervised areas should be identified in the local rules.

        True: Controlled areas and supervised areas must be clearly defined within an employer's local rules.

    c. The RPS is responsible for staff complying with local rules.

        True: The RPS is involved in many aspects of radiation protection, including investigating radiation overdoses, ensuring that staff follow local rules and carrying out investigations.

    d. Controlled and supervised areas should have a warning sign and indicate the nature of the hazard above the door.

        True: Clear warning signs are required to indicate controlled and supervised areas.

    e. Controlled and supervised areas are not required for mobile examinations.

        True: As mobile examinations are carried out in open wards or theatres, it would be impractical to designate the whole room as a controlled area because of the other people likely to be present. Normally a radiographer will designate a temporary controlled area of 2 m around the patient as the controlled area.

Q4.8 Radiation biology

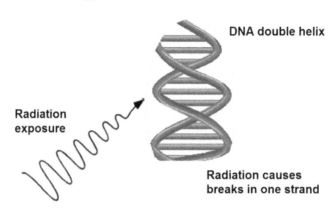

DNA double helix

Radiation
exposure

Radiation causes
breaks in one strand

The main impact of radiation (x- and gamma rays, electrons, beta and alpha particles) is that they cause ionization within the body. This ionization creates free radical molecules, mainly hydroxyl (OH), which is highly reactive and causes changes to DNA, RNA and other large molecules within the body. It should be noted that an ion and a free radical are not the same, as many ions react within the body in normal chemical reactions without any detrimental effect. A free radical is an atom or molecule that has one unpaired electron in its outer valence shell. It is well established in radiobiology that the more rapidly dividing a cell is the greater its radiosensitivity. The concept of lethal dose (LD) is used to indicate the dose of acute whole body radiation that causes death in 50% of the population exposed to it, within a period of time. For example, a dose of 4–5 Gy would create an LD of 50/30. This means that 50% of the population would be dead within 30 d of exposure.

Concerning radiation biology (true or false)
a. Common radiosensitive cells include spermatagonia, stem cells and lymph cells.
b. The primary cause of death due to radiation exposure is severe depletion of bone marrow stem cells.
c. Once exposed to radiation cells cannot recover.
d. Somatic effects are those that will affect the next generation.
e. Children are at greater risk than adults as they generally have longer to live.

Answers

   a. Common radiosensitive cells include spermatagonia, stem cells and lymph cells.

      True: These cells are at greater risk from radiation as they are rapidly dividing cells.

   b. The primary cause of death due to radiation exposure is severe depletion of bone marrow stem cells.

      True: Bone marrow is used as a good indicator of the degree of radiation damage.

   c. Once exposed to radiation cells cannot recover.

      False: Cells can be repaired after radiation damage and this complicates the setting of radiation exposures, as the body may be able to bear greater radiation exposure due to these repair mechanisms.

   d. Somatic effects are those that will affect the next generation.

      False: Somatic effects are those affect the individual, whereas genetic or hereditary effects are those that affect the next generation through mutagenesis.

   e. Children are at greater risk than adults as they generally have longer to live.

      True: This is one of the reasons why children are at greater risk of radiation damage. Another is that they have a greater number of rapidly dividing cells which are more radiosensitive.

Q4.9 Radiation safety of staff

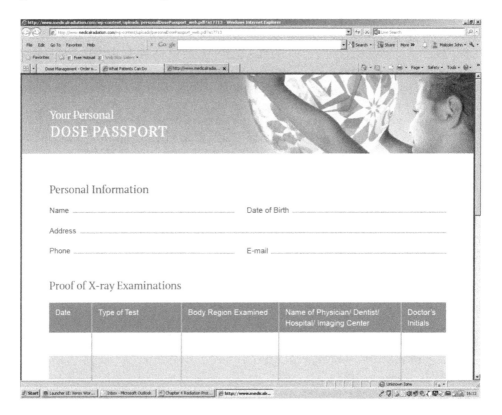

IRR (1999) and IRMER (2000) are used to guide and regulate exposure to patients and staff in the healthcare environment. The difference in the two regulations is that IRMER is concerned with exposures to patients whilst IRR addresses the radiation health and safety of staff. Different categories of staff are defined: referrer, practitioner and operator. The employer is responsible for record keeping, ensuring that education and training is up to date, and establishing referral and examination justification for radiation based examinations. Other duties include imaging protocols for each procedure, how to deal with pregnancy, assessment of patient dose and QA of equipment.

Concerning the safety of staff working with ionizing radiation (true or false)

 a. Dose limits are specified in IRR (1999).
 b. Exposure time and distance from radiation source are the best controls of radiation exposure to staff.
 c. Leakage radiation from the x-ray tube is the largest source of staff doses in fluoroscopy.
 d. Designated areas are defined to limit the probability and magnitude of a radiation accident.
 e. In fluoroscopy, staff dose rates tend to be lower when using an under-couch tube than when using an over-couch tube.

Answers

a. Dose limits are specified in IRR (1999).

True: These regulations are very much aimed at the employer and their responsibilities regarding radiation protection.

b. Exposure time and distance from radiation source are the best controls of radiation exposure to staff.

True: In fluoroscopy, techniques like image hold and pulsed exposures reduce the radiation exposure of staff. Using this along with the inverse square law are the best ways to reduce radiation. The next best technique is shielding, e.g. lead garments, gloves, drapes and eye/thyroid shields.

c. Leakage radiation from the x-ray tube is the largest source of staff doses in fluoroscopy.

False: There is leakage of radiation from the x-ray tube housing although it is only a few percent of overall operator exposure.

d. Designated areas are defined to limit the probability and magnitude of a radiation accident.

True: A controlled area is defined as one where staff have to follow special procedures to restrict significant exposure to ionizing radiation or prevent/limit the chance and scale of a radiation accident.

e. In fluoroscopy, staff dose rates tend to be lower when using an under-couch tube than when using an over-couch tube.

True: An under-couch tube reduces exposure to staff (via scatter radiation from the patient) and also to the operator's hands as hand exposure will occur after the beam has passed through the patient. However, the tube should not be positioned too close to the patient to minimize patient entrance dose.

Q4.10 Practical radiation exposure reduction

There are many practical ways of reducing radiation exposure without significant compromise of image or diagnostic quality.

Concerning reducing radiation exposure (true or false)

a. Changing the fluoroscopic frame rate from 25 fps to 12.5 fps will double the radiation dose to the patient.

b. The use of collimation will reduce the area of patient exposure and therefore dose.

c. A CT scan should never be performed on a pregnant patient.

d. A patient has received an 8 mSv dose from a nuclear medicine scan, therefore they cannot have a follow-up CT scan.

e. The dose to children visiting their parents after having a nuclear medicine examination must not be above 1 mSv.

Answers

a. Changing the fluoroscopic frame rate from 25 fps to 12.5 fps will double the radiation dose to the patient.

   False: Halving the frame rate should, ideally, halve the radiation dose (for the same kV, mAs settings) as there would be half the number of x-ray exposures.

b. The use of collimation will reduce the area of patient exposure and therefore dose.

   True: The smaller the area of the body exposed to radiation the lower the risk. This is also helped by a reduction in scatter radiation.

c. A CT scan should never be performed on a pregnant patient.

   False: A CT scan may be justified on a pregnant patient if the benefit outweighs the risk to the mother and foetus. It would obviously be prudent to use non-ionizing modalities such as US or MRI if possible.

d. A patient has received an 8 mSv dose from a nuclear medicine scan, therefore they cannot have a follow-up CT scan.

   False: Radiation doses from other examinations do not constrain the ability to use other modalities, the radiation risk is weighed up against the benefits of having the examination.

e. The dose to children visiting their parent after having a nuclear medicine examination may not be above 1 mSv.

   True: The limit of radiation exposure to a member of the public is 1 mSV per annum, regardless of their relationship.

Q4.11 Ionizing radiation dose I

Isotope	Application
Technetium 99m	Many applications including bone scans, ventilation scans, renograms and perfusion scans.
Iodine 131	Thyroid therapy
Iodine 123	Thyroid imaging
Thallium 201	Cardiology
Fluorine 18	PET scanning
Cobalt 60	Some forms of radiotherapy

It is conventional for a patient to receive a radiation exposure from a single source, but this is not always the case. Additional exposures may arise from different imaging procedures but may also occur when imaging supports therapy. This may occur when a patient attends for CT following a plain film x-ray or can occur when a patient attends for DEXA or perhaps spectral CT. Whilst a simple point to make, it is also often overlooked that a patient will receive a dose of radiation from environmental sources in addition to anything that is overseen medically.

Considering dose from multiple sources (true or false)
    a. If two radioactive sources are present, you only need to consider the dose from the higher activity source.
    b. The radiation field from effluent is never of consequence due to high dilution factors even though it may arise from a number of different diagnostic applications.
    c. Any staff member receiving an effective dose greater than 1 mSv automatically becomes a classified worker.
    d. IRR17 increased the threshold for classified workers from that in IRR99.
    e. The employer is legally bound to follow the advice of the appointed RPA.

Answers

a. If two radioactive sources are present, you only need to consider the dose from the higher activity source.

False: the dose from each must be calculated and it is the combination that is used to represent the dose, and hence risk, to the patient.

b. The radiation field from effluent is never of consequence due to high dilution factors even though it may arise from a number of different diagnostic applications.

False: There are strict limits on what can be released. This is enforced in England by the Environment Agency but all territories have similar controls in place.

c. Any staff member receiving an effective dose greater than 1 mSv automatically becomes a classified worker.

False: The 1 mSv limit is the limit for a member of the public. For a staff member the limit is 3/10 of the annual dose limit or 6 mSv. In practice, there would be an investigation before this limit is reached.

d. IRR17 increased the threshold for classified workers from that in IRR99.

False: The limit stayed the same. The limits for the eye and fingers was however decreased.

e. The employer is legally bound to follow the advice of the appointed RPA.

False: However, if the advice is not followed and there is patient detriment, then the consequences can be particularly severe.

Q4.12 Ionizing radiation dose II

The effect and consequences of ionizing radiation exposure on human biology is central to understanding the risk-benefit balance during patient investigations. This balance is not always as simple as it might first appear. Complexities might include repeated examinations, confirmed or suspected pregnancy or imaging paediatric patients. New techniques may also introduce the need for a more comprehensive understanding of risk than is the case for simple exams such as chest x-rays.

Regarding the types of dose (true or false)
- a. Neutrons have a radiation weighting factor that depends on their energy.
- b. The equivalent dose to the skin is measured in Gy because it is an organ.
- c. Although a non-ionizing technique, the risk from ultrasound can be summarised in radiation dose-equivalent terms.
- d. Thyroid dose from iodine is high because of the organ's propensity to collect iodine.
- e. The chemical toxicity of all materials is of secondary consequence to their radio toxicity.

Answers

   a. Neutrons have a radiation weighting factor that depends on their energy.

      True: The actual factor can be found in the usual references.

   b. The equivalent dose to the skin is measured in Gy because it is an organ.

      True: The effective dose is calculated by use of the tissue weighting factor and uses the unit, sievert, Sv.

   c. Although a non-ionizing technique, the risk from ultrasound can be summarised in radiation dose-equivalent terms.

      False: The risk from ultrasound has its own indicators that are totally different from those used in ionizing radiation and furthermore don't relate to fatal cancers.

   d. Thyroid dose from iodine is high because of the organ's propensity to collect iodine.

      True: The radioactive iodine locates preferentially in the thyroid, thus increasing the gland specific activity.

   e. The chemical toxicity of all materials is of secondary consequence to their radio toxicity.

      False: Chemical toxicity is always taken into account before its use is considered.

Q4.13 Safety in radiography I

The risks arising from imaging procedures can be complex and certainly extend beyond the familiar risk assessment from exposure to ionizing radiation. The premise of 'do no harm' is also impossible to achieve bearing in mind that any imaging technique requires an exchange of energy with the patient and heating, even if very minor, will always occur. A meaningful knowledge of imaging risks is crucial and apart from managing the best interests of the patient, not addressing any health detriment may lead to subsequent actions against the employer.

When considering sources of risk (true or false)

    a. The only relevant risk from x-ray imaging is that arising from the ionizing radiation.

    b. Contamination of the Technetium generator eluate in nuclear medicine is a risk to the patient.

    c. The risk to the driver delivering medical isotopes can be ignored because of the high level of screening built into delivery containers.

    d. MR conditional means that all medical devices can be taken into the imaging suite so long as conditions on the type of pulse sequence used are documented.

    e. Modern legislation links the risk indicators associated with ultrasound to be used for calculating patient health detriment.

Answers

a. The only relevant risk from x-ray imaging is that arising from the ionizing radiation.

> **False:** In fact there are numerous risks such as that from the use of contrast agents, electrical safety.

b. Contamination of the Technetium generator eluate in nuclear medicine is a risk to the patient.

> **True:** There are strict requirements to ensure sterility is maintained and that there are no other contaminants such as molybdenum breakthrough.

c. The risk to the driver delivering medical isotopes can be ignored because of the high level of screening built into delivery containers.

> **False:** There is strict legislation to ensure that the goods are carried and looked after properly. This includes how to manage accidents and security. The packaging has to be sufficiently robust and also attenuating to ensure the driver is not exposed to ionizing radiation that could elevate his exposure above the statutory limits.

d. MR conditional means that all medical devices can be taken into the imaging suite so long as conditions on the type of pulse sequence used are documented.

> **False:** MR conditional means that there must be a special case made to ensure that the device is safe and the patient is unlikely to be harmed. The term conditional refers to the scan has been approved conditional on those safety measures being in place.

e. Modern legislation links the risk indicators associated with ultrasound to be used for calculating patient health detriment.

> **False:** The ultrasound risk indicators do not directly relate to a measurable risk to the patient—they provide an indication of the increase or decrease of an effect occurring but not what that probability actually is.

Q4.14 Safety in radiography II

Whilst risk to the patient forms a significant part of the management of imaging techniques, the risks to attendant staff must also be properly addressed. By definition staff will receive a small radiation dose for every patient exposure and hence the aggregate to the staff member may be significant over time with appropriate concerns over health detriment. The management of staff risk can be complex especially where staff rotate through different modalities.

Regarding risk to employees (true or false)
    a. Pregnant staff are obliged to wear electronic dose meters that alarm when a threshold dose has been reached.
    b. Film badges are now banned from use in staff dose surveys.
    c. Thermoluminescent dosimeters (TLDs) can be affected by exposure to high magnetic fields and hence must not enter the MRI suite.
    d. Hormesis is a well-established concept that modifies the risk factor from ionizing radiation at low doses.
    e. When using isotopes in gaseous form, room ventilation is an important factor in staff dose-reduction.

Answers

   a. Pregnant staff are obliged to wear electronic dose meters (EPDs) that alarm when a threshold dose has been reached.

      False: Staff are obliged to be monitored but how this is done will vary with local protocols. Some staff will value the additional reassurance that EPDs provide but there is no obligation.

   b. Film badges are now banned from use in staff dose surveys.

      False: they can still be used but they are less sensitive and far less convenient to use than the current thermoluminescent dosimeters (TLDs), optical luminescent dosimeters (OLDs) or electronic dosimeters.

   c. Thermoluminescent dosimeters (TLDs) can be affected by exposure to high magnetic fields and hence must not enter the MRI suite.

      False: TLDs are ceramic in nature and are not affected by magnetic fields. However, the equipment necessary to readout and process them is not MR compatible.

   d. Hormesis is a well-established concept that modifies the risk factor from ionizing radiation at low doses.

      False: Hormesis relates to the possible variation of risk with low dose and in some models even suggests that there might be a net benefit to very low radiation exposures. This is counter to the currently used best understanding using the Linear No Threshold Model.

   e. When using isotopes in gaseous form, room ventilation is an important factor in staff dose-reduction.

      True: The radioactive gas exhaled by a patient will contribute to the occupational exposure of the staff member. This can be considerable when aggregated over a number of patients and must be taken into account in room design and occupancy factors.

Q4.15 Safety in radionuclide imaging I

Components of Bio-medical waste (Cont...)

Components	Examples
▪ Soiled waste	• Dressing, bandages, plaster casts, material contaminated with blood
▪ Chemical waste	• Alcohol, Sulphuric acid, chlorine powder, Glutaraldehyde, Picric acid, fertiliser, ammonia
▪ Discarded medicines and cytotoxic drugs	• Barium enema, X-rays, Cancer chemotherapy, tar-based products
▪ Radioactive Components ▪ Incineration ash	• EtBr, Radioactive components

The creation of waste in hospitals is commonplace, however, some radiological techniques create waste with a radioactive component. This radioactive waste introduces additional considerations for radiation protection and associated additional legislation and guidance from the Environment Agency. The production and management of radioactive waste is important to understand.

With regard to the management of waste (true or false)
a. Departments where isotopes are used must employ the services of a Radiation Waste Advisor (RWA).
b. There is a significant risk to the environment from radioactive waste disposal.
c. The cremation of patients having recently undergone brachytherapy is banned as a result of the release of radiation to the atmosphere.
d. Dilution factors are important when calculating environmental risk assessments.
e. Dressings from radioactive patients are unlikely to present a radiological risk.

Answers

a. Departments where isotopes are used must employ the services of a Radiation Waste Advisor (RWA).

True: This is a complex area of environmental protection and the RWA is now a statutory appointment in a similar manner to the RPA.

b. There is a significant risk to the environment from radioactive waste disposal.

True: However, care is taken to ensure that any radioactive waste disposed of to the environment falls within strict limits.

c. The cremation of patients having recently undergone brachytherapy is banned as a result of the release of radiation to the atmosphere.

False: There are guidelines that relate to the cremation of patients with implants such as pacemakers and radioactive seeds. It is important that the relevant department is notified of such implants so that the appropriate calculations can be made. It may be the case that implants are removed if the cremation is delayed.

d. Dilution factors are important when calculating environmental risk assessments.

True: If the dilution of a released isotope is great enough, the exposure to a member of the public will be very low.

e. Dressings from radioactive patients are unlikely to present a radiological risk.

False: They can present a risk where the absorbed body fluid has a significant radioactive presence. It is usually the case that departments using radioactive materials with patients have a radioactive store to allow any body fluids to decay before disposal.

Q4.16 Safety in radionuclide imaging II

Radiation exposure to staff can arise from a variety of mechanisms. This includes to the hands of operators when drawing up radioactive drugs to syringes. Monitoring of finger doses is important particularly to reduce risk to the staff member but also to ensure good practice is being adhered to and to reduce such doses below that embedded in legislation and guidance.

In relation to physical risk (true or false)
   a. Syringe shields are used to minimise the radiation risk to the staff member's whole body.
   b. Well counters are used to ensure the activity given to the patient falls within the limits contained within the Administration of Radioactive Substances Advisory Committee (ARSAC) documentation.
   c. Any isotope spillage is unlikely to be of consequence due to the low volumes used.
   d. Radiation protection guidelines require all waste to be isolated to reduce staff exposure.
   e. Finger doses are more likely to be raised than eye doses.

Answers

a. Syringe shields are used to minimise the radiation risk to the staff member's whole body.

False: they are used to reduce finger dose. There is an implication for the staff member's effective dose, but if the radiation field was large enough to present a direct whole body risk, then other methods of protection would be used.

b. Well counters are used to ensure the activity given to the patient falls within the limits contained within the Administration of Radioactive Substances Advisory Committee (ARSAC) documentation.

True: well counters are specially configured ion chambers which are designed to record the radiation emitted in almost all directions. They therefore produce an accurate readout of the activity in the syringe.

c. Any isotope spillage is unlikely to be of consequence due to the low volumes used.

False: any spill will elevate the exposure to surrounding staff, patients or visitors. The exposure may not be large but is in excess of what is normally expected and hence must be controlled.

d. Radiation protection guidelines require all waste to be isolated to reduce staff exposure.

True: any source of radiation must be considered for control, by isolation or removal.

e. Finger doses are more likely to be raised than eye doses.

True: in nuclear medicine there are many occasions where manual handling of radioactive sources is necessary. Even using syringe shields and the familiar time, distance and shielding principle, finger doses are usually slightly higher than in other areas using ionizing radiation.

Q4.17 Radionuclide radiation protection

The needs of the patient define their treatment and whilst this is an almost universal statement, there are some aspects of how the patient is managed that are complex. The radiation effects on the patient, family members of the patient and members of the public who might come into contact with them need to be considered. There are many difficulties in calculating these risks, since the exact movements of the patient are uncertain as is the proximity of those who might be affected, but guidelines do exist to ensure that any dose that is given to the patient or other incidental individuals is estimated.

When managing of patients (true or false)
a. Iodine ablation patients are usually kept in hospital overnight because otherwise they might cause an excess dose in those around them.
b. There is no need for isolated toilet facilities for use by nuclear medicine patients since the biological half-life is so long.
c. Patient jewellery can be the origin of artefacts in ventilation perfusion (VQ) scans.
d. Single photon emission computed tomography scanners often have proximity detectors to prevent any untoward contact between the patient and the scanner.
e. The ideal half-life for an imaging isotope is as short as possible to ensure a low dose to the patient.

Answers

a. Iodine ablation patients are usually kept in hospital overnight because otherwise they might cause an excess dose in those around them.

> **True:** The activity required to cause the required therapeutic effect is sufficient for the patient to be significantly radioactive into the following day. The patient is monitored until their activity falls below a level that is likely to cause a threshold exposure to family members or other individuals in proximity to them.

b. There is no need for isolated toilet facilities for use by nuclear medicine patients since the biological half-life is so long.

> **False:** patient waste will be sufficiently radioactive to introduce a risk to the environment if not properly managed. This is an important role of the RPA and RWA.

c. Patient jewellery can be the origin of artefacts in ventilation perfusion (VQ) scans.

> **True:** dense material such as metallic jewellery can attenuate the gamma rays and be visible on the image. The same is true of garments such as bras.

d. Single photon emission computed tomography scanners often have proximity detectors to prevent any untoward contact between the patient and the scanner.

> **True:** Scanners such as SPECT have the best performance when in very close proximity to the patient. There is a risk that the scanner could collide with the patient and hence a proximity or contact device is included to avoid patient harm.

e. The ideal half-life for an imaging isotope is as short as possible to ensure a low dose to the patient.

> **False:** Whilst a short half-life can reduce the exposure to the patient, it also makes the imaging very difficult and may also prevent the adequate localisation of the carrier pharmaceutical. A rough approximation is that the effective half-life should be similar to the duration of the study.

IOP Publishing

Scientific Basis of the Royal College of Radiologists Fellowship (2nd Edition)

Illustrated questions and answers

Malcolm Sperrin and John Winder

Chapter 5

Computed tomography

The introduction of CT revolutionised imaging in that it provided high resolution tomographic imaging (the production of images that represent slices of tissues). This also meant that the visualisation of anatomy presented challenges since most imaging previously had been projection based leading to overlying tissues appearing coincident on the final image. CT was previously known as Computerised Axial Tomography (CAT) scanning since the original imaging systems had a gantry which only allowed for axial reconstruction of images. The advent of spiral CT and 3D reconstruction also means that the association with axial scanning is largely redundant with the gantry angle now being selectable to minimise partial effects or to minimise radiation dose. Despite the advances of new imaging techniques within CT, it does present challenges associated with the increased radiation dose and there are commercial drivers that encourage asymptomatic screening that controversially elevates radiation dose without obvious benefit.

Q5.1 Computed tomography back projection

High contrast object back projected onto image matrix

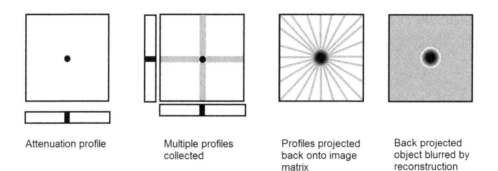

| Attenuation profile | Multiple profiles collected | Profiles projected back onto image matrix | Back projected object blurred by reconstruction |

In CT scanning the x-ray tube is pulsed on and off (for a few milliseconds) whilst the gantry on which the tube is held rotates around the patient. Each pulse of x-rays is attenuated as it passes through the patient and a profile of the x-ray attenuation is collected by the bank of detectors on the opposite side of the gantry. The linear attenuation profiles are combined and reconstructed into an image using a technique called back projection. The figure shows the steps in the back projection process and how a single high contrast object is formed after imaging.

Concerning CT image reconstruction (true or false)
    a. Filtered back projection can give rise to a star artefact.
    b. The iterative technique is much faster than filtered back projection.
    c. Digital filtration is used to sharpen the resultant image.
    d. A bow tie filter is used to enhance sharpness.
    e. Data interpolation is used in helical CT scanning to reconstruct images.

Answers

    a. Filtered back projection can give rise to a star artefact.

        True: Attenuation profiles recorded from around the patient are mapped back onto the image matrix and lead to the start artefact.

    b. The iterative technique is much faster than filtered back projection.

        False: The iterative technique uses an approximation model to the CT image and then takes multiple mathematical steps (iterations) to achieve a full image.

    c. Digital filtration is used to sharpen the resultant image.

        True: Digital filtration can smooth or edge enhance an image. In the case of CT, edge enhancement is used to reduce the impact of the star artefact introduced in the reconstruction process.

    d. A bow tie filter is used to enhance sharpness.

        False: The bow tie filter is a used to change the intensity profile of the x-ray fan beam so that less radiation is used at the edges of the patient and more is used at the centre where the patient attenuates x-rays the most. It results in improved CT image uniformity and number accuracy.

    e. Data interpolation is used in helical CT scanning to reconstruct images.

        True: Data acquisition in helical CT is not from a single plane but is recorded on a spiral pathway. To obtain a planar CT image (as opposed to one that is non-planar), data interpolation is used to calculate what the attenuation would be at a given point between two rotations.

Q5.2 Technology in cone beam computed tomography

Cone beam CT (CBCT) uses a beam of x-rays that is similar in configuration to a conventional x-ray set. The beam is cone shaped and exposes a volume of tissue rather than on a slice basis as in conventional CT. CBCT acquires hundreds of planar images (analogous to the x-ray attenuation profiles collected in CT). The x-ray beam is pulsed to reduce radiation exposure and CBCT creates radiation doses up to 10 times smaller than conventional CT. The data acquisition time is relatively short, however, volume reconstruction time is of the order of minutes. It has high resolution (less than 0.1 mm) and a low effective dose (30–500 μSv) compared to conventional CT, which may be a few millisieverts.

Concerning CBCT (true or false)
    a. An entire volume of (three-dimensional) data is generated in one gantry rotation.
    b. CBCT is capable of higher spatial resolution compared to multislice CT (MSCT).
    c. CBCT has a gantry rotation time similar to MSCT of 1.0 s.
    d. X-ray scatter is a degrader of image quality.
    e. Scatter in CBCT results in the cupping artefact and streaking.

Answers

   a. An entire volume of (three-dimensional) data is generated in one gantry rotation.

   True: CBCT uses an x-ray beam that is shaped like a cone and a flat panel detector using caesium iodide (doped with thallium) of dimensions 40×30 cm. The whole detector is exposed continuously during the 360° rotation.

   b. CBCT is capable of higher spatial resolution compared to MSCT.

   True: The detector matrix in CBCT is of the order of 2048×1500, producing voxel sizes of 200 µm, whereas MSCT would typically produce a voxel size of 600 µm. Both systems are capable of higher spatial resolution, however, this requires much greater x-ray exposure and is not routine.

   c. CBCT has a gantry rotation time similar to MSCT of 1.0 s.

   False: For a C-arm CBCT the gantry rotation time is between 5–20 s depending on other acquisition parameters.

   d. X-ray scatter is a degrader of image quality.

   True: As the cone beam has greater physical dimensions than a fan beam, scatter becomes much more significant. There are no anti-scatter septae in the cone beam detector and therefore scatter remains a problem.

   e. Scatter in CBCT results in the cupping artefact and streaking.

   True: The scatter to primary beam ratio for MSCT is about 0.2, whereas it is much greater for CBCT at 3.

Q5.3 The cone beam effect in computed tomography scanning

The cone beam effect is a potential source of image artefacts, especially in the more peripheral regions of the scan volume. The amount of data corresponds to the total amount of recorded attenuation along a specific beam projection angle as the scanner completes the rotation. The total amount of information for peripheral structures is reduced because the outer row detector pixels record less attenuation, whereas more information is recorded for objects projected onto the more central detector pixels. This results in image distortion, streaking artefacts and greater noise in the peripheral region. This effect is minimized by manufacturers incorporating various forms of cone beam reconstruction. Clinically, it can be reduced by positioning the region of interest adjacent to the horizontal plane of the x-ray beam.

Concerning the cone beam effect (true or false)
   a. The fan beam in MSCT diverges in the z-direction to a greater extent than single slice CT.
   b. The greater the divergence of the x-ray beam the lower the cone beam effect.
   c. The cone beam effect is greater for 16 slice scanners compared to four slice scanners.
   d. Detectors in the middle of the cone beam suffer from less cone beam effect than those at the detector outer edges.
   e. The cone beam effect can lead to artefacts at the upper and lower edges of the image volume.

Answers

a. The fan beam in MSCT diverges in the z-direction to a greater extent than single slice CT.

True: The detector size in MSCT is greater than in single slice CT along the z-direction. This means that less collimation is used in MSCT. Also, the fan beam in single slice CT is collimated by tungsten jaws both at the x-ray tube and also at the detector.

b. The greater the divergence of the x-ray beam the lower the cone beam effect.

False: As the divergence of the cone beam increases more of the body is irradiated that is outside the intended location of a particular slice and therefore the greater the potential contribution of data to the slice.

c. The cone beam effect is greater for 16 slice scanners compared to four slice scanners.

True: Off axis objects are 'seen' or projected onto different detectors' rows during a rotation, leading to mis-registration of data.

d. Detectors in the middle of the cone beam suffer from less cone beam effect than those at the detector outer edges.

True: In figure B the cone beam effect shows that the data acquired from outer detectors are not on a single plane.

e. The cone beam effect can lead to artefacts at the upper and lower edges of the image volume.

True: Data collected by detectors come from the area of overlap of the beam as it rotates around the patient. At the outer edges of the beam the overlap is greater due to the angle of the beam at the edges which increases the area of overlap. The wider the cone angle the greater the potential for artefacts. Artefacts can be reduced by improved reconstruction algorithms.

Q5.4 Principles of computed tomography operation

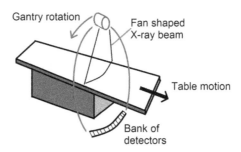

A helical CT scanner collects a volume of data whilst the patient is continuously moved through the scanner gantry. This results in a spiral exposure path around the patient and x-ray linear attenuation profiles are collected that are not exactly on the same slice plane. New image reconstruction techniques are required with data interpolation providing the mechanism to produce a 'flat' or planar slice of anatomy. Helical CT has evolved using multiple row detectors to collect data and reconstruct multiple slices from one rotation of the gantry. This shortens examination time but also enables a new range of examinations so the increased use of CT will increase population dose even if individual subject dose does not change.

In helical CT (true or false)
- a. Image quality is affected by the pitch.
- b. Increasing the bore diameter will reduce image resolution.
- c. Image reconstruction can only be achieved following a minimum rotation of 360°.
- d. Image acquisition time is limited by the duration of the tube rotation around the patient.
- e. Radiation exposure increases in proportion to pitch factor.

Answers

a. Image quality is unaffected by the pitch.

False: Pitch is defined as the distance of table movement divided by the collimator width. As pitch is increased in helical CT, for the same mAs and kV, image noise will increase and the partial volume effect may be accentuated, although image contrast would be largely unaffected.

b. Increasing the bore diameter will reduce image resolution.

False: Increasing the bore diameter makes the size of the detector larger but the angle over which it accepts data will be unaffected other than the fact that more scatter might reduce the contrast.

c. Image reconstruction can only be achieved following a minimum rotation of 360°.

False: All points must be sampled in order to obtain an image and this can equally be performed by rotating through 180°. This is an important concept since for very large pitch factors, tissue will not be sampled through 360° and an image is formed even if image quality and artefacts may start to become a consideration.

d. Image acquisition time is limited by the duration of the tube rotation around the patient.

True: The image will be constructed as the tube rotates. If the tube rotates quickly then the image will be formed faster but the noise will increase because the amount of time each detector is acquiring data will be reduced.

e. Radiation exposure increases in proportion to pitch factor.

False: Large pitch factors reduce the amount of radiation administered to the patient since the scanned volume will be covered faster.

Q5.5 Multislice detectors in computed tomography

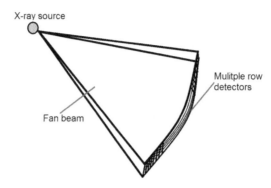

One of the most significant developments in CT in recent years is the development of multiple row detectors. Previously, one linear attenuation profile was recorded for each rotation of the CT gantry. With multidetector CT a broader fan beam exposes rows of detectors which enable multiple slices to be collected in a gantry rotation. A broader slice of tissue is exposed and the table motion is much more rapid to prevent overlapping exposures (although this is a technique used for cardiac applications, resulting in a pitch value of less than 1.0). Manufacturers of CT scanners may define pitch differently, some take number of slices per rotation into account.

Concerning multidetector CT (true or false)
- a. The limiting resolution for slice thickness is defined by the detector element size.
- b. Scintillating ceramics provide low afterglow in detecting x-rays.
- c. A patient scanned with a 5 mm slice, at a table speed of 10 mm s^{-1} and a rotation time of 1 s results in a pitch of 1.5.
- d. Data from multiple detector rows may be averaged together to reduce noise and slice thickness.
- e. The efficiency of the detectors is unaffected by the detector septa size.

Answers

a. The limiting resolution for slice thickness is defined by the detector element size.

   True: Multislice detectors may have row sizes of 0.5 mm or 0.6 mm. This is the minimum slice thickness that could be achieved with this type of detector. It is rarely used due to the level of noise present in such a thin slice.

b. Scintillating ceramics provide low afterglow in detecting x-rays.

   True: Ceramics have good x-ray absorption and produce light proportional to the incident x-ray photons. There is very little afterglow from these detectors compared to older gas types.

c. A patient scanned with a 5 mm slice, at a table speed of 10 mm s^{-1} and a rotation time of 1 s results in a pitch of 1.5.

   False: Pitch = table speed/slice thickness for one rotation and these parameters would give a pitch of 2.

d. Data from multiple detector rows may be averaged together to reduce noise and slice thickness.

   False: Data from multiple detector rows are averaged together with a subsequent reduction in noise, however, this results in thicker slices rather than thinner slices.

e. The efficiency of the detectors is unaffected by the detector septa size.

   False: Each individual element of a multiple row detector is surrounded by a septa which makes it distinct from its neighbouring element. The septa material does not contribute to the detection of x-rays and therefore contributes to the inefficiency of the detector.

Q5.6 Spatial resolution in computed tomography

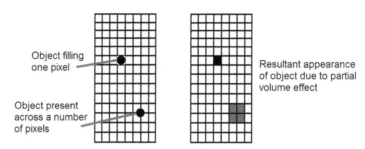

Object filling one pixel

Object present across a number of pixels

Resultant appearance of object due to partial volume effect

The spatial resolution of a CT scanner is dependent on a number of factors. The number and size of the individual detector elements, the slice thickness (which affects resolution in the z-direction), the x-ray tube focal spot size, the reconstruction algorithm, the image matrix and the FOV. Spatial resolution is measured in line pairs per centimetre or millimetre and test objects offer pairs of materials that have very different linear attenuation to provide the line pairs. Note that even a high contrast object that is detected in a number of pixels due to its position will have its inherent contrast reduced as the signal is spread between the pixel values. This is an example of the partial volume effect in the image matrix. This also occurs, more significantly, in the z-direction (greater slice thickness results in diminution of contrast).

Spatial resolution in CT (true or false)
   a. Is typically $5\,\mathrm{lp\,mm}^{-1}$ for a head CT.
   b. Is greater than in digital mammography.
   c. Can be increased with the use of iodine based contrast media.
   d. Can be described as isotropic for a voxel of dimensions $0.5 \times 0.5 \times 0.5\,\mathrm{mm}$.
   e. Has a pixel size of 1.6 mm for a 40 cm FOV.

Answers

a. Is typically $5\,lp\,mm^{-1}$ for a head CT.

   False: If the image matrix is the limiting factor in spatial resolution, the resolution can be estimated using the formula 1/(pixel size $\times$ 2), since we need two pixels to resolve an object. Therefore, the pixel size in head CT is ~0.47 mm (240 mm FOV/512), spatial resolution = 1/(0.47 $\times$ 2) = $1.07\,lp\,mm^{-1}$.

b. Is greater than in digital mammography.

   False: Digital mammography has the highest spatial resolution of all x-ray based modalities with a value of $20\,lp\,mm^{-1}$.

c. Can be increased with the use of iodine based contrast media.

   False: Contrast media will not affect the spatial resolution of an imaging modality, but will affect the contrast resolution.

d. Can be described as isotropic for a voxel of dimensions $0.5 \times 0.5 \times 0.5$ mm.

   True: The definition of an isotropic voxel is that its sides are of equal dimensions.

e. Has a pixel size of 1.6 mm for a 40 cm FOV.

   False: A pixel size is defined as the FOV/image matrix. 400 mm/512 = 0.781 mm.

Q5.7 Computed tomography image reconstruction

Step 1	Make an intial estimate of the image
Step 2	Calculate attentuation profiles based on this image
Step 3	Compare to acquired projections
Step 4	Use difference to update original image

Iterative reconstruction is an old technique making a comeback for the reconstruction of medical images from raw data. The iterative technique differs from the conventional filtered back projection in that it starts with a 'guess' image and deconstructs the individual projections from that image. These projections are then compared to the real projections (acquired during scanning) and it uses a statistical model to determine the noise present and seeks to reduce this. This technique takes more time computationally, but produces images less sensitive to noise and produces better quality images when not all the raw data are available.

Concerning CT image reconstruction (true or false)
   a. The movement of the gantry enables profiles of linear attenuation to be recorded.
   b. The profile sampling is generally more frequent than every 0.5° or rotation.
   c. Hounsfield units are based on the attenuation of x-rays to bone.
   d. The fan beam is defined by the x-ray tube output window.
   e. In helical CT the image plane is reconstructed using interpolation.

Answers

a. The movement of the gantry enables profiles of linear attenuation to be recorded.

True: As the CT gantry rotates around the patient, the x-ray tube is pulsed on and off and a profile of linear attenuation is measured through the patient each time the x-ray beam is pulsed on.

b. The profile sampling is generally more frequent than every 0.5° or rotation.

True: Depending on the scanner there may be up to 1000 profiles recorded in one 360° rotation, which means more frequently than every 0.5°.

c. Hounsfield units are based on the attenuation of x-rays to bone.

False: The Hounsfield unit scale is based on knowing the linear attenuation of water and each measurement (for tissues) is compared to this.

d. The fan beam is defined by the x-ray tube output window.

False: The fan shaped x-ray beam in CT is defined by tungsten or steel collimators near the x-ray tube and also in front of the detector back.

e. In helical CT the image plane is reconstructed using interpolation.

True: As the raw data (x-ray attenuation profiles) are acquired along a helical pathway as the patient is driven through the gantry, the plane from which these profiles are recorded is not flat but distorted. To reconstruct an image in a plane that is perpendicular to the table movement direction (transverse slices), data interpolation is required. This means 'estimating' a new attenuation coefficient between two measured points.

Q5.8 Computed tomography image presentation

The measurement of x-ray linear attenuation is converted into the Hounsfield scale and pixel values are called Hounsfield units or CT numbers. They have a range of 4096 (−1024 to +3072) and are calibrated against water which has a CT number of zero. As there are normally 256 grey levels available to us on a computer monitor, if the grey levels are allocated across the CT number range equally we may lose a lot of detail in the image (each grey level would represent 16 CT numbers). Therefore some subtle differences in x-ray attenuation may be allocated the same grey level and be indistinguishable. If we focus the allocation of grey levels to a specified range (many bodily tissues have CT numbers in the range −100 to +100), we can visualize differences between tissues as small as one CT number.

Concerning image display in CT (true or false)
   a. A typical image matrix is 128×128.
   b. Decreasing the window width (WW) increases overall image contrast.
   c. The CT number window centre (WC) indicates the range of pixel values across which the grey scale is allocated.
   d. A setting of $WW = 1000$ and $WC = -500$ would be useful for visualizing the mediastinum.
   e. Reformatted images have the same spatial resolution regardless of the image plane.

Answers

a. A typical image matrix is 128×128.

   False: CT has an image matrix of 512×512 for routine display for all areas of the body. However, images may be interpolated and presented as 1024×1024.

b. Decreasing the WW increases overall image contrast.

   True: Decreasing the WW reduces the number of grey levels and has the impact of increasing contrast between tissues.

c. The CT number WC indicates the range of pixel values across which the grey scale is allocated.

   False: The WC (sometimes called window level) defines the pixel value to which the middle grey level is allocated. The CT number range over which the grey scale is allocated is known as the WW.

d. A setting of $WW = 1000$ and $WC = -500$ would be useful for visualizing the mediastinum.

   False: As the WC is -500 the middle grey value is allocated to very low density tissues, those containing air perhaps. The width of 1000 indicates that the grey level range from black to white is from 0 to -1000. This window setting is more likely to be used to visualize the lungs.

e. Reformatted images have the same spatial resolution regardless of the image plane.

   False: Reformatted images are those generated from the reconstructed transverse images. If isotropic voxels are used then the spatial resolution in the x-, y- and z-directions will be the same. However, most routine scans have a slice thickness (z size) greater than the pixel dimension (x and y) and therefore the resolution will differ depending on which direction is considered.

Q5.9 Computed tomography

Iterative Reconstruction
Pathway

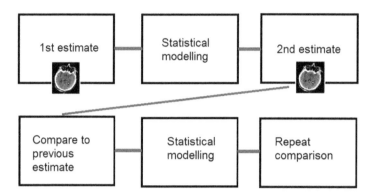

In computed tomography, images are reconstructed from linear attenuation profiles. Iterative reconstruction can improve the image quality, however, is computationally more expensive, requiring faster computing power. Iterative reconstruction begins with a basic CT image calculated by the filtered back projection technique. It then models the original attenuation profiles and reconstructs a new image which is compared to the original. This cycle is repeated until the difference in images reaches a preset value. Iterative reconstruction is useful in routine imaging to reduce noise but has also found application in the reduction of metal artefacts and in cardiac imaging where attenuation profiles are damaged or missing.

In CT image reconstruction (true or false)
    a. Filtered back projection produces images with fewer artefacts than iterative reconstruction.
    b. Iterative reconstruction produces images of lower noise than filtered back projection.
    c. Iterative reconstruction is a slower computation method than filtered back projection.
    d. The implementation of iterative reconstruction may result in dose reduction to patients.
    e. Iterative reconstruction results in a smoother image.

Answers

a. Filtered back projection produces images with fewer artefacts than iterative reconstruction.

   False: Iterative reconstruction can reduce noise, streak artefacts and metal artefacts.

b. Iterative reconstruction produces images of lower noise than filtered back projection.

   True: Iterative reconstruction has the potential to reduce noise by using mathematically modelled attenuation profiles (which have very low noise content).

c. Iterative reconstruction is a slower computation method than filtered back projection.

   True: Iterative reconstruction requires multiple steps which may be repeated many times and therefore is computationally expensive.

d. The implementation of iterative reconstruction may result in dose reduction to patients.

   True: Yes, reduced noise is possible and therefore the mAs may be reduced accordingly, in selected scanning techniques.

e. Iterative reconstruction results in a smoother image.

   True: Reduced noise will result in less grainy images and therefore these would be perceived as smoother.

Q5.10 Computed tomography radiation dose

Dose length product = $CTDI_{vol}$ x scan length

where $CTDI_{vol}$ is
the CT dose index

Dose length product is
measured in mGy.cm

As computed tomography has continued to develop, the effective dose has reduced. There are several factors for this, including improved detector efficiency, improved beam filtration, and automatic exposure control systems. Better selection of CT scanning parameters and limitation to the CT scanning range have contributed to reduced effective dose. Scan protocols should be designed to achieve the minimum image quality required for the specific investigation, rather than aiming for high image quality for all techniques. New methods such as CT fluoroscopy and dynamic CT are inherently high dose techniques. They require high spatial resolution and low noise and generate high numbers of images.

Radiation dose in computed tomography is dependent on (true or false)
   a. The mA and kVp settings of the x-ray tube.
   b. The body mass of the patient.
   c. The radiation detector efficiency.
   d. The length of the anatomy being scanned.
   e. The body composition of the patient.

Answers

   a. The mA and kVp settings of the x-ray tube.

       True: Yes, the tube current and voltage potential settings have a significant impact on radiation received by the patient.

   b. The body mass of a patient.

       True: Increased body mass of the patient will require increased radiation. More x-ray photons will be scattered or absorbed in a larger patient and these will not contribute to image formation. Therefore, for a larger patient for whom a given image quality is to be maintained, the mAs must increase.

   c. The radiation detector efficiency.

       True: Yes, the more efficient the radiation detector, the less radiation will be required for the same noise content.

   d. The length of the anatomy being scanned.

       True: The greater the anatomical range scanned, the greater the radiation dose (increased mAs).

   e. The body composition of the patient.

       True: In abdomen/pelvic CT, the adipose content has a significant bearing on the overall radiation dose.

Q5.11 Spectral computed tomography

Computed tomography generates images based on the linear attenuation coefficient of tissues, averaged across the energies contained within the x-ray spectrum. Spectral CT, also known as dual energy CT, has emerged recently as a technique which measures the linear attenuation coefficients of tissues at two separate energies (for example, 80 kVp and 120 kVp). This technique exploits the fact that the attenuation of x-rays for one tissue differs at these two energies. This means that through image subtraction, tissue types can be separated more easily, for example contrast enhanced blood vessels (iodine) and bone (calcium).

Concerning spectral (multi-energy) computed tomography (true or false)
    a. Utilises the difference in linear attenuation coefficients between materials at two different x-ray tube kilovoltage settings.
    b. X-ray tube energy ranges from 20 kVp to 45 kVp.
    c. Two x-ray tubes sit opposite each other on the gantry.
    d. The tube voltage may be rapidly switched between low and high energy.
    e. Is used to separate iodine contrast agent from bone.

Answers

a. Utilises the difference in linear attenuation coefficients between materials at two different x-ray tube kilovoltage settings.

True: Conventional single tube/energy CT uses the tissue attenuation averaged across the tube x-ray spectrum. Spectral CT aims to exploit the differences in attenuation at different x-ray energy.

b. X-ray tube energy ranges from 20 kVp to 45 kVp.

False: Typical x-ray tube energies would be between 60 kVp and 140 kVp.

c. Two x-ray tubes sit opposite each other on the gantry.

False: Spectral CT scanners may have two separate x-ray tubes at two different energies positioned at right angles to each other.

d. The tube voltage may be rapidly switched between low and high energy.

True: x-ray tubes are capable of being switched rapidly between 100 kVp and 140 kVp which aids near simultaneous acquisition of low and high energy data.

e. Is used to separate iodine contrast agent from bone.

True: One of the strengths of spectral CT is its ability to differentiate between materials of different atomic number, for example, iodine and calcium.

IOP Publishing

Scientific Basis of the Royal College of Radiologists Fellowship (2nd Edition)

Illustrated questions and answers

Malcolm Sperrin and John Winder

Chapter 6

Ultrasound

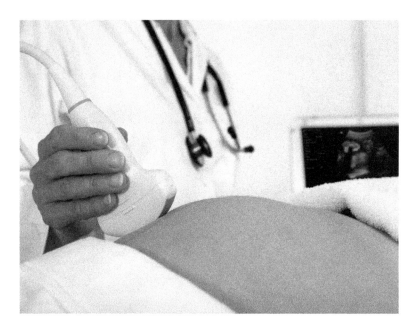

Ultrasound provided a revolution in medical imaging since its initial introduction in the 1970s. It is generally accepted as being very low risk mainly as a result of it utilising non-ionizing radiation to form the image. However, it also has the benefit of being essentially real-time with a frame rate that can be considered to freeze motion of the heart. It is also very useful in that it can measure blood flow without recourse to interventional techniques and combine this information within an anatomical image. There are very many ultrasound options some of which enhance tissue contrast, others enable the creation of highly specialist transducers which combine to establish a diverse and efficacious modality. The small size also makes the use of ultrasound in the community a realistic proposition although this does create some problems since image interpretation can be a challenge.

Q6.1 Ultrasound imaging: routine

Diagnostic US is routinely used in cardiac, obstetric, musculoskeletal and paediatric investigations. US a not an EM radiation as it is uses sound waves which do not possess enough energy to be ionizing. The main reported hazards associated with US are heating, streaming and cavitation. The heating effect is used in therapeutic ablation applications of US. Streaming is a mechanical response of cells to the US beam passing through and is manifest as movement of the cells along lines coincident with the US beam shape. Cavitation is the interaction of the US waves with microbubbles with the body, potentially leading to increase in bubble size and subsequent damage to tissue. Cavitation requires continuous high intensity US energy unlikely to be encountered in diagnostic examinations.

Concerning routine diagnostic abdominal US (true or false)
    a. Only qualified radiologists are permitted to use the image for diagnostic purposes.
    b. There are no practical limits on US exposure.
    c. High US frequencies are used to reduce risk to the patient.
    d. Some patients correctly report being able to hear the US.
    e. The risk indicators thermal index (TI) and mechanical index (MI) are measures of the probability of tissue damage.

Answers

a. Only qualified radiologists are permitted to use the image for diagnostic purposes.

   False: This can be quite a contentious issue. Many professional groups utilize US for diagnostic purposes. Such professional groups include radiologists, radiographers, rheumatologists, physiotherapists, medical physicists, etc. Most employers require the user of the US to follow protocols and demonstrate their competence by certification and on-going training.

b. There are no practical limits on US exposure.

   False: Most professional bodies and sometimes national legislation put a limit on the exposure to US. This is usually a function of time and power although the overlying premise is the minimum exposure required to ensure the benefit to the patient is realized. This is different from the exposure to ionizing radiation where limits are clear and exceeding them must be fully justified.

c. High US frequencies are used to reduce risk to the patient.

   False: Frequencies are not selected according to their risk. The choice of frequency is usually driven by the need for spatial resolution. There may be some confusion here since the penetration of the US is reduced at higher frequencies meaning that the US energy is absorbed in a smaller volume which leads to a higher potential temperature rise. However, whilst this may be true, this is picked up by the TI.

d. Some patients correctly report being able to hear the US.

   False: This is impossible for two reasons. First, the ear is not sensitive to frequencies in the MHz range and second US will not propagate through air sufficiently to reach the ear of the patient. The strong reflection at solid–air boundaries also makes any propagation to the patient of very low intensity. What the patient may hear is the electrical trigger giving the pulse repetition rate of a few kHz which does fall within the audible range.

e. The risk indicators MI and TI are measures of the probability of tissue damage.

   False: These two indicies are mathematical constructs which vary with mechanical and thermal bioeffects, respectively. They are parameters which may be used as threshold indicators above which damage may occur, therefore they are not directly related to risk.

Q6.2 Ultrasound imaging: obstetrics

A major application of diagnostic US is in obstetrics where it is used for a variety of applications from gestational age determination to anomaly scanning. Whilst being a non-ionizing modality, the technique still propagates energy into the patient and foetus and effects such as heating are known to occur and some observers postulate athermal effects, although this is highly contentious and there is no convincing evidence of such effects being relevant to the health of the patient. The use of Doppler is different in that some applications rely on the US being used to insonate a small volume for extended periods. Different manifestations of Doppler do exist, such as duplex, power and spectral Doppler, each having its own specialist use. One common misconception is that Doppler is an imaging technique. This is not really the case—Doppler is a mathematical explanation of a frequency shift which can be used to colour certain parts of the image but by itself is not an imaging technique.

In obstetric scanning (true or false)
    a. Particular care needs to be taken during insonation of a foetus in the first trimester.
    b. Doppler techniques are used in order to reduce risk to the foetus.
    c. Power Doppler can be used to identify flow direction.
    d. US image formation time is too long to permit control by cardiac gating.
    e. Transvaginal techniques are used to improve image quality.

Answers

a. Particular care needs to be taken during insonation of a foetus in the first trimester.

True: The first trimester is the time during which any challenge to the foetus is most risky. Whilst no evidence exists that relates US to foetal risk, it is still prudent to limit any exposures, especially since future understanding of bioeffects may reveal currently unknown mechanisms of damage.

b. Doppler techniques are used in order to reduce risk to the foetus.

False: In fact the opposite is true since Doppler is usually considered to be a high intensity technique. Doppler is chosen once the area to be studied is imaged and then only used as necessary following the normal best guidance. Doppler as an option is chosen to reveal blood flow information and is non-invasive, leading to less trauma for sensitive patient groups. Doppler can be used to obtain data that are otherwise unavailable such as pulsatile profiles.

c. Power Doppler can be used to identify flow direction.

False: Power Doppler integrates the intensity of the returning Doppler shifted frequencies. The integration process leads to a signal that reflects the amount of shift rather than actual shifted frequency and hence is a crude measure of number of scatterers which is in turn related to blood flow volume. This is a useful technique where flow volume may be low and hence determining the very low shifted frequencies that provide information about direction may be noisy and difficult to interpret. Combining all of the shifted frequencies will give an indication of small flow volumes and be of use where perfusion may be uncertain such as in tumours or transplants.

d. US image formation time is too long to permit control by cardiac gating.

False: The frame rate possible with modern scanners and transducers runs into many hundreds. This means that you can obtain an image at a precise moment in the cardiac cycle and the QRS complex can be used to trigger the image acquisition process.

e. Transvaginal techniques are used to improve image quality.

True: Intracavity probes enable the transducer elements to get closer to the target area of interest. The reduced penetration means that higher frequencies can be used and hence image quality, especially resolution, is improved. There are other considerations that will inform the user such as the vital need for electrical safety and elevated heating effects.

Q6.3 Ultrasound imaging: image process

US can be considered to be an imaging modality that uses tissue acoustic properties to be the basis of contrast. There are many subtleties which contribute to the appearance of the final image and also the creation and control of the acoustic wave make US very user dependent. A comprehensive knowledge of the physical processes behind the technique will permit greater use to be made. US is also prone to numerous artefacts, some of which may be useful in the diagnostic process and an understanding of their origin is helpful especially if such artefacts are a limiting factor in the image quality.

Concerning US (true or false)
  a. Resonance considerations prevent a given transducer crystal emitting off-frequency.
  b. The acoustic impedance of bone makes intra-joint imaging prohibitively difficult.
  c. M-mode imaging cannot be used to provide anything other than qualitative information.
  d. Absorption is the primary mechanism of intensity reduction.
  e. MI values are tissue specific.

Answers

a. Resonance considerations prevent a given transducer crystal emitting off-frequency.

   False: Resonance is a physical property that is used to enhance the conversion of electrical energy into acoustic energy. The resonance referred to is the natural frequency of vibration being matched to the driving frequency which means in turn that less electrical energy is required to create a given intensity. The transducer element will still oscillate if driven off-resonance but its vibrational amplitude will be reduced and more of the electrical energy will dissipate as heat.

b. The acoustic impedance of bone makes intra-joint imaging prohibitively difficult.

   True: The acoustic impedance step from soft tissue to bone creates a very large reflection coefficient meaning that there is insufficient propagation to form an image. There are specialist techniques using small or specially shaped probes that permit imaging in joint spaces but such techniques are very specialist and may not be available in many US departments.

c. M-mode imaging cannot be used to provide anything other than qualitative information.

   False: M-mode utilizes the movement of boundaries to form an image and is often used for cardiac studies where the bright echo that signifies the presence of a boundary of a heart valve (for instance) will move and form a characteristic line. Structures that move quickly will show different patterns to those that move slowly and similar arguments apply to the amplitude of the motion. It is possible to analyse the image to obtain structural information but it is also used as a qualitative information.

d. Absorption is the primary mechanism of intensity reduction.

   True: US can be scattered, absorbed or reflected but all transmission has absorption associated with it even if reflection or scatter do not occur. There will clearly be occasions when the imaged volume is so small that almost all US is reflected rather than absorbed, but for most imaging, absorption is dominant.

e. MI values are tissue specific.

   False: TI is dependent on the tissue being insonated since the thermal properties of tissue and how they convert acoustic energy into thermal energy will also depend on tissue type. In the case of MI, the risk is more associated with the onset of cavitation which is less dependent on tissue type and more dependent of the presence of gas bubbles.

Q6.4 Ultrasound imaging: transducer

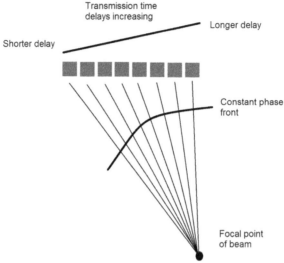

The US transducer is central to the formation of the image and its use, design and potential faults will significantly affect the final image. Transducer design has evolved over the years from single element transducers which are now rarely encountered to highly complex phased arrays and intracavity transducers which have specialist applications. How the transducer works is also core knowledge since it affects the resolution and bioeffects.

Concerning general US technique (true or false)
 a. Phased arrays are primarily used for their ability to generate high frame rates.
 b. Trans-oesophageal echo can be used to create high frame rate cardiac images.
 c. Superficial tissue heating is solely due to heat conduction from the transducer.
 d. Lateral resolution can be controlled by the user.
 e. Axial resolution is a function of ultrasonic pulse length.

Answers

a. Phased arrays are primarily used for their ability to generate high frame rates.

   False: The high frame rate is one benefit of the phased array but there are other attributes which are just as important. They provide for a finer focus and also are much smaller than other options such as linear arrays. Apart from cardiac studies, it is the ability to form high quality images rather than high frame rates that is of prime importance.

b. Trans-oesophageal echo can be used to create high frame rate cardiac images.

   True: The use of trans-oesophageal echo means that the separation between transducer and target volume can be reduced. This has two consequences: first, because the penetration distance is reduced, a higher frequency can be used and second, because the echo return time is lower, the frame rate can increase.

c. Superficial tissue heating is solely due to heat conduction from the transducer.

   False: Being electrical, some of the energy will be transformed into heat within the transducer which can become warm. However, heating also arises from the absorption of acoustic energy and these are two of a number of heating causes.

d. Lateral resolution can be controlled by the user.

   True: The lateral resolution can most easily be thought of as being related to the beam width. Reducing the beam width will improve spatial resolution since it reduces the separation of features that can be resolved. Whilst there is a beam width that is dependent on the transducer architecture, you can also reduce the beam width by focusing the beam using the delays on the transducer elements.

e. Axial resolution is a function of ultrasonic pulse length.

   True: Axially, the resolution is governed by the length of the transmitted pulse which is typically three or four wavelengths.

Q6.5 Harmonic imaging I

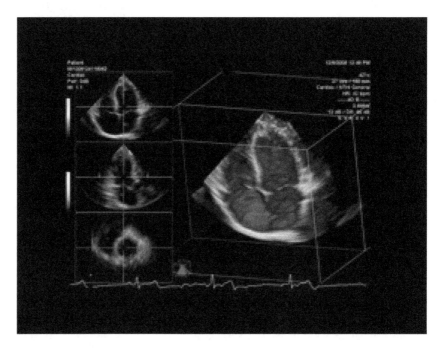

Harmonic imaging is a relatively recent option but one that is a significant aid to improving image quality. It relies on the tissue through which the US is travelling having different properties during high and low pressure sections of the wave. This makes the wave more complex in shape and a mathematical analysis reveals this to be a complicated combination of a number of waves rather than just the original transmitted wave. How this complex wave is reflected, detected and displayed forms the basis of harmonic imaging.

Concerning harmonic imaging (true or false)
1. Harmonic imaging utilizes the variation in acoustic velocity with the pressure that varies with the passage of the ultrasonic wave.
2. Acoustic velocity increases with pressure.
3. The returning echo comprises two or more discrete waves.
4. Use of the harmonic imaging option improves the image quality at depth.
5. Harmonic imaging will alter the TI and MI risk indicators.

Answers

a. Harmonic imaging utilizes the variation in acoustic velocity with the pressure that varies with the passage of the ultrasonic wave.

True: Waves propagate faster in high pressure environments than low. This means that the positive part of the wave will try to catch up with the low pressure part of the wave leading to a saw-tooth appearance.

b. Acoustic velocity increases with pressure.

True: At low pressures, the effect on velocity is small but as the pressure increases, the variation between high and low pressure velocity increases.

c. The returning echo comprises two discrete waves.

True: The evolution of the complex wave can be mathematically described by the superposition of two or more waves at different frequencies and phases. The easiest way to think of this is a room full of talking people each of whom has a voice of a certain frequency and who starts talking at a different time and hence the phases are different too. The combined effect is to create a complicated sound comprising the many different components.

d. Use of the harmonic imaging option improves the image quality at depth.

True: Because you select to use the wave at a higher frequency, the resolution is improved, but the wave has an origin deep within the tissue and hence has a shorter distance to travel thus resulting in a reduced attenuation. This improves the SNR and contrast.

e. Harmonic imaging will alter the TI and MI risk indicators.

False: Whilst you choose to eliminate the fundamental frequency for use in the image reconstruction, the full multitude of frequencies is still in place and hence any bioeffects will still be present.

Q6.6 Acoustic field

US imaging relies on the creation of an acoustic field which is reflected or scattered by the tissue through which it passes. The shape and extent of this field has a critical role in key aspects of the image such as spatial resolution and beam width and hence a working knowledge of the factors affecting the field shape is important.

Concerning the acoustic field (true or false)
    a. A small transducer element behaves as a point source.
    b. Large transducer elements give rise to a large near field.
    c. The near field is alternatively known as the Fraunhofer zone.
    d. A useful approximation of the imaging depth is 100 wavelengths.
    e. Focused transducers act to reduce the beam width.

Answers

a. A small transducer element behaves as a point source.

True: For a source of US to act as a point source, it must be smaller than a wavelength. This means that the element must typically be less than about 0.5 mm and probably much smaller than this. For a phased array of 2 cm and containing 128 elements, the transducer size is 0.15 mm or smaller and hence the individual elements will behave as point sources.

b. Large transducer elements give rise to a large near field.

True: The extent of the near field is calculated by the simple equation; distance = aperture diameter^2/wavelength. The near field is therefore proportional to transducer element size squared.

c. The near field is alternatively known as the Fraunhofer zone.

False: An alternative name for the near field is the Fresnel Zone. This is a historical consideration.

d. A useful approximation of the imaging depth is 100 wavelengths.

True: This is a useful approximation derived from tissue attenuation properties, SNR, etc.

e. Focused transducers act to reduce the beam width.

True: A focal point is simply where the acoustic energy is preferentially directed. This means that the beam width is also reduced.

Q6.7 Thermal index and mechanical index

Obstetric Scanning

US is accepted to be a very low risk imaging modality. At diagnostic intensities, there are few if any reports of induced harm to the patient but prudent practice dictates a cautious approach by the operator. Two known potential bioeffects are heating and cavitation and all modern scanners are required to display risk indicators based on these risks. A general guide to safety supported by most professional bodies requires the exposure time to be reduced and the risk indicators to be minimized.

Concerning the safety of US
a. The TI is subdivided to reflect the heating of certain tissue types.
b. A TI of 0.5 represents half the risk of a TI of 1.0.
c. The MI is independent of frequency.
d. Acoustic intensity is a major factor in both TI and MI.
e. Absolute limits apply to TI used for obstetric scanning as a result of the risk to the foetus.

Answers

   a. The TI is subdivided to reflect the heating of certain tissue types.

      True: The thermal properties of tissue vary with tissue type, perfusion and also their proximity to strongly reflecting features such as bone surfaces. For this reason the temperature elevation is calculated according to one of three options: soft tissue, bone and cranial. The user needs to ensure that the correct TI is selected for reporting.

   b. A TI of 0.5 represents half the risk of a TI of 1.0.

      False: This is a common misconception. The risk indicators are used to reveal a trend in risk when other imaging parameters are changed. Hence increasing power will increase the TI, but it does not reveal what happens to the risk to the patient. This is a clinical judgement since a damage threshold may be approached which is not reflected in the TI value.

   c. The MI is independent of frequency.

      False: The frequency is taken into account, appearing as its square root as the divisor. This means that as the frequency is increased, the MI value will decrease but not linearly. This does make sense since for a bubble to grow and collapse, a certain time is required which may be too short for high frequencies.

   d. Acoustic intensity is a major factor in both TI and MI.

      True: Intensity will increase the temperature and local pressures.

   e. Absolute limits apply to TI used for obstetric scanning as a result of the risk to the foetus.

      False: The TI is an indicator of risk and not a measure of it. Whilst good practice does recommend limits, it is the clinical need that is the primary driver.

Q6.8 Image formation

US images comprise a succession of lines of US which themselves contain information about the acoustic path followed. The presence of echoes is indicative of acoustic impedance changes in the exposed tissue, the size of which can be used to infer information about the echogenicity of the tissue boundary itself. This physical manifestation of the tissue properties can be used to good purpose by the sonographer.

Concerning the formation of the image (true or false)
    a. Acoustic impedance is the product of frequency and wavelength.
    b. The lungs are difficult to image due to almost complete reflection from the tissue boundary.
    c. Time gain control can be used to compensate for intensity loss arising from scatter, absorption and reflection.
    d. The frame rate is independent of the line density.
    e. The image is brightest at shallow depths solely as a result of skin being very echogenic.

Answers

a. Acoustic impedance is the product of frequency and wavelength.

False: This equation gives the velocity. Acoustic impedance is the product of density and velocity and takes either the appropriate SI unit or the unit rayl. It is easy to confuse the two equations.

b. The lungs are difficult to image due to almost complete reflection from the tissue boundary.

True: It is the echo reflected from boundaries that is used as the basis of the image. If there is sufficient reflection from a boundary to prevent any significant US to propagate beyond the boundary, then no image will be formed. This is the basis for acoustic shadowing.

c. Time gain control can be used to compensate for intensity loss arising from scatter, absorption and reflection.

True: As US propagates through tissue the wave intensity is reduced as a result of attenuation arising from absorption scatter and reflection. Instead of applying amplification at all depths which would amplify those depths where attenuation is not significant, it is possible to amplify according to depth. This is known as depth gain compensation or time gain compensation.

d. The frame rate is independent of the line density.

False: The US image comprises a series of adjacent lines each containing the echoes from a particular direction. Each line represents the passage of the outgoing and returning echo so the total time to form the image is the product of the number of lines and the time taken to form one line, hence fewer lines lead to a higher frame rate.

e. The image is brightest at shallow depths solely as a result of skin being very echogenic.

False: The image is brightest partly because of a strong reflection from the skin boundary but also because the US has the greatest intensity which gives rise to the strongest echoes.

Q6.9 Artefacts

Conventional Imaging   Fatty Tissue Imaging

Artefacts are a feature of any imaging system and can be a limiting factor in the diagnostic potential. The precise nature of the artefact will depend upon the physics of the imaging process and hence an understanding of the origin and nature of an artefact can provide insight into how it can be reduced, eliminated or even utilized for diagnosis. There are many artefacts in US and their recognition is an important aspect of the training programme.

Concerning artefacts you might encounter in an image (true or false)
    a. Comet-tail artefacts arise from localized highly attenuating material.
    b. Refraction artefacts are associated with 'scatterers' smaller than a wavelength.
    c. Reverberation artefacts can be associated with poor acoustic coupling to the patient's skin.
    d. Acoustic shadowing is an artefact that can be utilized in imaging through the bladder to view a foetus.
    e. Uroliths are too small to give rise to artefacts.

Answers

   a. Comet-tail artefacts arise from localized highly attenuating material.

      False: The artefact arises because the enhanced attenuation reduces the amount of US penetrating beyond the given region. Because there is less US, the returning echoes will therefore be darker than those adjacent to the region of interest, giving the appearance of a dark streak behind the material. This is shadowing and is the opposite of the comet tail artefact.

   b. Refraction artefacts are associated with 'scatterers' smaller than a wavelength.

      False: Refraction occurs where the US path is modified by the presence of a specular reflector at non-orthogonal incidence. The US may therefore be reflected by objects not on the original transmitted path and will therefore appear in the wrong location. Small 'scatterers' give rise to Rayleigh scattering which does not permit the formation of an image.

   c. Reverberation artefacts can be associated with poor acoustic coupling to the patient's skin.

      True: This artefact occurs when there is very high reflection from a boundary which causes the US to bounce back and forward from the transducer to the skin surface a number of times before eventually decaying away. One common reason for the strong reflection from the skin is poor application of coupling gel.

   d. Acoustic shadowing is an artefact that can be utilized in imaging through the bladder to view a foetus.

      False: The full bladder can act as a low attenuation window to the developing foetus making imaging less prone to artefacts and poor image quality. The full bladder has few 'scatterers' and hence has reduced attenuation. It is associated with being a comet tail artefact, which is where an enhanced acoustic energy arises deeper than the foetus giving rise to a bright region as opposed to the dark region caused by the acoustic shadowing.

   e. Uroliths are too small to give rise to artefacts.

      False: Uroliths have a density and acoustic velocity generally higher than the surrounding soft tissue making the reflection coefficient large. This results either in a strong reflection and hence an acoustic shadow, or a significant scatter, again reducing the intensity propagating beyond it.

Q6.10 Bioeffects

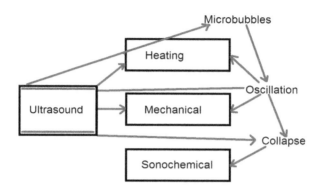

All imaging processes rely on an interaction of energy with tissue and hence are associated with a bioeffect. Such bioeffects may be of vanishingly small relevance but they must be identified since they may become significant if developments lead to increased intensities. There are likely to be many effects that affect the potential well-being of the patient all of which will be different in nature and severity and the crucial skill is to be able to identify the risk, reduce its impact and maintain the diagnostic potential of the technique. Being non-ionizing, US is not associated with the same risks as x-rays, but nevertheless studies have shown that risks do exist and need to be managed.

Concerning bioeffects (true or false)
    a. Heating is the primary concern at diagnostic intensities.
    b. Cavitation is a risk that is enhanced during the use of contrast agents.
    c. The ability of the patient to dissipate heat is a factor in the consideration of risk.
    d. Patients correctly correlate risk with the audible sound from the transducer.
    e. Stasis is a common risk.

Answers

a. Heating is the primary concern at diagnostic intensities.

True: Any energy entering the body will partly give rise to heating. In the extreme case, if all of the US is attenuated then it will all contribute to heating. However, it is important to put this in context since whilst the risk is real, the actual temperature rise is small and only under certain circumstances would the temperature elevation be of concern.

b. Cavitation is a risk that is enhanced during the use of contrast agents.

True: Cavitation is a process where a small bubble grows under the repeated positive and negative cycling encountered by tissue during insonation. The bubbles can either be naturally present in tissue or under extreme circumstances can form in response to very low pressures in the same way as bubbles form when removing the top of a bottle of fizzy drink. The contrast agents which are themselves bubbles are therefore a cavitation risk.

c. The ability of the patient to dissipate heat is a factor in the consideration of risk.

True: The human body is efficient at transporting and regulating temperature. Where such thermoregulation is compromised or when the temperature challenge is excessive, then the local temperature rise can be of concern.

d. Patients correctly correlate risk with the audible sound from the transducer.

False: What patients can hear is the line refresh triggers in the transducer which are often in the audible range. Ultrasonic frequencies are well beyond the audible range and US does not propagate readily through air.

e. Stasis is a common risk.

False: Stasis is where the force that arises from a travelling wave is sufficient to move or prevent movement in blood. This may occur in fine capillaries but good practice ensures that the transducer is kept moving or that the transmitted power is zero when the image is frozen, making stasis a possibility but also unlikely.

Q6.11 Contrast agents

US imaging can suffer from poor contrast and this can be a limiting factor for its use in some key potential applications. For instance, the acoustic impedance step across blood vessels may be insufficient for them to be imaged even though the limit of resolution has not been reached. Techniques do exist for enhancing contrast which utilize the physical properties of the travelling wave.

Concerning contrast agents (true or false)
 a. Commonly used contrast agents have typical dimensions of less than 5 µm.
 b. Being gas-filled, contrast agents have a high reflection coefficient.
 c. The enhanced reflection is the primary mode of operation of agents.
 d. Contrast agents are very short lived which limits their use to cardiac applications.
 e. Dispersion in the blood is a known complication of the use of contrast agents.

Answers

a. Commonly used contrast agents have typical dimensions of less than 5 µm.

True: This is important since it permits the ready passage of the agent through capillary networks and also the bubbles will act as small scatterers leading to contrast enhancement from harmonic propagation of the reflected US.

b. Being gas-filled, contrast agents have a high reflection coefficient.

True: However, they may not exist in sufficient numbers to make a whole area have increased contrast as a result of the increased reflection coefficient. Contrast agents also permit the use of harmonic techniques, making their action derived from two mechanisms.

c. The enhanced reflection is the primary mode of operation of agents.

False: The concentration of the agents is sufficient to make them enhance contrast but their use in harmonic imaging is now generally thought to be of the primary benefit.

d. Contrast agents are very short lived which limits their use to cardiac applications.

False: The agents are relatively short lived but their admission to the blood stream is designed to enhance cardiac imaging. Such agents would have benefit at other sites of interest such as the liver, but traditionally the agent lifetime means that any effect is marginal. However, agents are being developed with longer useful lifetimes which introduce the possibility of contrast enhanced imaging of sites other than the heart.

e. Dispersion in the blood is a known complication of the use of contrast agents.

True: Contrast agents can disperse via a number of mechanisms including solution and also clumping. Clumping can lead to occluded vessels as the agents are designed to dissolve relatively quickly. Whilst this is a complication that limits their use, it is also a convenient safety mechanism.

Q6.12 The Doppler effect

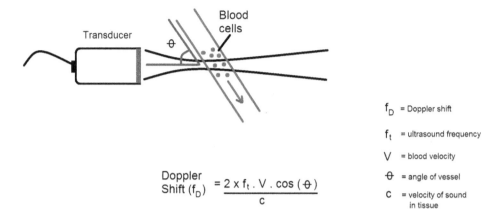

f_D = Doppler shift

f_t = ultrasound frequency

V = blood velocity

θ = angle of vessel

C = velocity of sound in tissue

$$\text{Doppler Shift } (f_D) = \frac{2 \times f_t \cdot V \cdot \cos(\theta)}{c}$$

The use of the Doppler effect in US is now well recognized. It was revolutionary in that it permitted functional information to be displayed against a background of anatomical information which made diagnosis easier for a number of conditions. Prior to the use of Doppler, quantitative blood flow measurements were difficult, if not impossible. The Doppler effect can be exploited to provide both qualitative and quantitative information, but it is associated with certain difficulties which makes its use challenging.

Concerning the Doppler effect (true or false)
a. Depth information can only be obtained by using continuous wave Doppler.
b. Aliasing is a limiting factor when using pulsed Doppler to measure high blood velocities.
c. The factor of two in the Doppler equation arises as a result of two Doppler path lengths.
d. Doppler can only be used to measure peak velocities.
e. Doppler shifts can only be recorded if the angle of insonation is known.

Answers

   a. Depth information can only be obtained by using continuous wave Doppler.

      False: Accurate depth information can only be derived from timing a returning pulse. Continuous wave Doppler does not use discrete pulses and so it contains no accurate time of flight information that can be used to determine depth.

   b. Aliasing is a limiting factor when using pulsed Doppler to measure high blood velocities.

      True: In order to determine the frequency shift, the US wave form must be analysed by sampling it. A wave can be unambiguously measured if more than two samples are taken for each wave cycle. In the simplest case, each transmitted line of US will sample the shifted wave and hence there must be two US lines transmitted for each shifted wave. This gives a limit to the shifted wave frequency for a given line refresh rate.

   c. The factor of two in the Doppler equation arises as a result of two Doppler path lengths.

      True: Because the transducer acts as transmitter and receiver and it is the reflector that is moving, there is a shift as it propagates and another as it returns giving the factor of two in the equation.

   d. Doppler can only be used to measure peak velocities.

      False: Any moving reflector will generate a Doppler shift. Where blood is moving all with the same velocity, only one shift will be generated and this could be thought of at the familiar wave profile. For lower velocities such as at the edge of vessels, the velocity giving rise to the shift will appear as in-fill below the envelope of the profile of the waveform.

   e. Doppler shifts can only be recorded if the angle of insonation is known.

      False: Doppler shifts can be recorded under many circumstances, but a knowledge of the insonation angle permits the user to calculate the blood velocity from the Doppler shift.

Q6.13 Power Doppler

Applications of Doppler US are extensive. New applications are continuously developing and one such development is power Doppler. This does not display the shifted frequency but rather displays the total shifted power from any Doppler shifted frequency. This is related to the volume of scatterers giving rise to the Doppler shift and hence is a useful indication of perfusion rather than simply the velocity of the flow.

Concerning power Doppler (true or false)
    a. Power Doppler requires knowledge of the insonation angle.
    b. Very small velocities can be used to contribute to the overall power Doppler signal.
    c. Pulsatile motion from vessel walls is irrelevant in the display of the Doppler signal.
    d. Power Doppler can be used to quantify blood flow volumes.
    e. Power Doppler can be useful in determining the efficacy of transplants.

Answers

a. Power Doppler requires knowledge of the insonation angle.

False: Power Doppler is simply a representation of the total amount of shifted US rather than the calculated velocity and hence there is no requirement to determine the insonation angle.

b. Very small velocities can be used to contribute to the overall power Doppler signal.

True: Because the power Doppler image utilizes the total shifted frequencies rather than discrete velocities, even very low Doppler shifts will be included in the overall calculation. This is one of the benefits of the technique since it is possible to determine low volume flow rates such as in transplants where colour flow imaging would struggle. There will still be a point below which you try to image noise but such thresholds are very low.

c. Pulsatile motion from vessel walls is irrelevant in the display of the Doppler signal.

False: If it moves, then there will be a derived Doppler signal. There is a facility called wall-thump filtration which analyses the Doppler signal in terms of its pulsatility and recognizes the wall thump as being associated with the passage of the blood pulse, rather than the velocity of the blood itself. This can be processed out of the data that are used to form the colour flow image or spectral Doppler trace.

d. Power Doppler can be used to quantify blood flow volumes.

True: Because it uses all shifted frequencies, it represents total blood movement and not that associated with particular velocities.

e. Power Doppler can be useful in determining the efficacy of transplants.

True: Being sensitive to low flow rates, the technique can be used in applications such as transplant assessment.

Q6.14 Duplex Doppler

Radial Artery

The overlaying of Doppler information on a two-dimensional grey scale image is conventionally known as colour flow imaging or duplex scanning. The ability to associate a given position with blood flow information is useful when assessing obstructions in vessels, flow rates from organs and foetal blood flow as well as numerous other examples. The accuracy of display of a Doppler signal is crucial both in terms of its location and velocity, and careful testing is performed to ensure that the complex image is suitable for use.

Concerning duplex Doppler (true or false)
    a. Colour flow imaging associates a colour to a direction of blood flow.
    b. The insonation angle is determined automatically by the location of the signal within the image.
    c. Colour flow information cannot be displayed in real time.
    d. Turning on colour flow will significantly reduce the resolution.
    e. Turbulent flow can appear as a complex pattern or as a green hue.

Answers

   a. Colour flow imaging associates a colour to a direction of blood flow.

      True: The returning US wave is mathematically interrogated to reveal the amplitude and direction of flow. This is displayed over the grey scale image to reveal of pattern of colours that is indicative of flow direction which is of considerable diagnostic value.

   b. The insonation angle is determined automatically by the location of the signal within the image.

      False: The insonation angle and also the width of the gate from which the US is to be analysed is selected by the user. In colour flow imaging the signal is recorded from a point which the computer system can calculate and hence an indicative velocity scale is shown, but for spectral Doppler this has to be selected.

   c. Colour flow information cannot be displayed in real time.

      False: The display does have a very short delay which arises from the time taken to process the US echoes and then display the image and overlaying colours, but it is considered to be real time.

   d. Turning on colour flow will significantly reduce the resolution.

      False: The resolution of the image will not change and is a function of pulse length and beam width. The resolution of the colour overlay will also not change since it is derived from the frequency shift of the returning echoes.

   e. Turbulent flow can appear as a complex pattern or as a green hue.

      True: The presence of turbulent flow will generate small changes in the flow pattern that the system will find difficult to associate with a given position. There will be positive and negative shifts which the system will correlate to turbulence and will be shown as green to differentiate it from predominantly laminar flow.

Q6.15 Harmonic imaging II

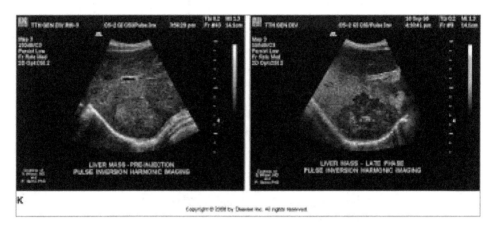

Harmonic imaging is a relatively new technique that utilizes the manner in which US propagates through tissue. The basic principle is that the acoustic velocity is dependent on local pressure and hence the positive pressure part of the wave propagates faster than the negative part, leading to a divergence from a pure sine wave. The mathematical description of this distorted wave relies on the fact that it can be represented by a succession of sine waves at successively higher multiple frequencies but reduced intensities. This does not mean that there is a multitude of waves propagating but rather the wave is simply no longer a pure sine wave. It requires a mathematical analysis once detected by the transducer for the higher frequency information to be extracted and displayed.

Concerning harmonic imaging (true or false)
 a. The harmonic image utilizes waves of increased resolving power.
 b. Harmonics form at increased depths.
 c. The technique can be used to reduce image noise.
 d. Resolution is improved over the fundamental image.
 e. Contrast agents also display harmonic enhancement.

Answers

    a. The harmonic image utilizes waves of increased resolving power.

        True: The non-linear propagation of the wave generates harmonics and the first harmonic is selected for use in the image. The first harmonic has twice the fundamental frequency and therefore has a greater associated resolution which is one of the benefits of this technique.

    b. Harmonics form at increased depths.

        True: The principle behind the technique is that the velocity of the wave is pressure dependent. This means that the longer the wave travels, the greater will be the difference between the faster and slower elements of the wave. This implies that the wave's distortion increases with time and therefore also distance.

    c. The technique can be used to reduce image noise.

        True: The SNR within the image will depend upon the signal size as well as the general random background noise. The speckle pattern will be frequency dependent with a lowering of noise as the frequency increases because the type of scattering will change as wavelengths decrease.

    d. Resolution is improved over the fundamental image.

        True: The frequency of the wave used for harmonic image is twice that of the image based on the fundamental frequency. If you remove the fundamental, the frequency used is increased and hence the resolution associated with that frequency is also increased.

    e. Contrast agents also display harmonic enhancement.

        True: Being encapsulated gases, contrast agents are very non-linear in their response to the US wave. The contrast agents therefore act in two ways: first, they are effective at the generation of harmonics and second, they are strong reflectors.

Q6.16 Transducer design

The US transducer is a vital component in ultrasonic imaging. Each component has a specific and important role which, if absent, will affect the functionality and hence use of the transducer. Transducers do degrade and it is important to be clear when a feature in the image is as a result of device failure in order to maximize image quality and reduce risk to the operator and patient. All transducers share certain common elements and differences often arise from scale and repetition rather than variance in core design.

Concerning transducer design (true or false)
    a. The small size of the elements in a phased array means the emitted US can be considered to be a continuous wave front.
    b. The crystal element is typically one wavelength thick.
    c. The backing layer reduces the transmitted pulse length.
    d. Trans-oesophageal probes present particular risks from electrical leakage.
    e. Imaging transducers cannot be used for colour flow imaging.

Answers

a. The small size of the elements in a phased array means the emitted US can be considered to be a continuous wave front.

True: Huygens principle states that if a transmitter is small enough it can be considered as a point source. The size at which this becomes a reasonable approximation is a wavelength. For a phased array of 2 cm containing 128 elements, this makes each element no larger than 0.16 mm. For a 3 MHz transducer, the wavelength is 0.5 mm which means that up to about 10 MHz the transducer can be considered to contain elements acting as point sources.

b. The crystal element is typically one wavelength thick.

False: For the element to be most efficient, it needs to resonate. The resonance will occur at multiples of half a wavelength and as the thickness increases it will be less efficient so a half wavelength is generally used.

c. The backing layer reduces the transmitted pulse length.

True: If the transducer element is activated by the electrical pulse and then allowed to listen, the element will continue to ring in the same way as the tone from a struck piano string continues to sound even when the hammer is removed. This continuing vibration will be confused with the returning echoes so a backing layer is applied to the crystal to prevent this ringing.

d. Trans-oesophageal probes present particular risks from electrical leakage.

True: Being so close to the heart, any electrical problems with the probe are potentially critical. Also, all of the transducer will be in contact with patient (rather than just the transmitting surface) and hence there is a greater chance of any transducer damage being present also being in contact with the patient.

e. Imaging transducers cannot be used for colour flow imaging.

False: Colour flow information is derived from the shift of the returning echoes. The echoes are used for two purposes, imaging and shifted frequency, and the technique is hence called Duplex.

Q6.17 Improving the image

The contrast and resolution that can be associated with an US image is known to be dependent on the user. A comprehensive knowledge of the underlying physics will permit the user to identify those actions that might lead to an image of improved diagnostic potential. Furthermore, some patients present challenges as a result of their size or volumes of gas which make obtaining an image particularly challenging. Increased penetration can result from increasing the acoustic power, but this also increases the risk indicators which is contrary to best practice.

Concerning actions to improve the image (true or false)
    a. Additional penetration may be achieved by the use of a lower frequency.
    b. Aliasing of the pulsed Doppler signal can be eliminated by decreasing the scan depth.
    c. Increasing the frequency only increases resolution in a harmonic image.
    d. Turning on Doppler imaging will reduce the frame rate.
    e. Improving the image by the use of multiple focal zones has no effect on the frame rate.

Answers
  a. Additional penetration may be achieved by the use of a lower frequency.
     True: US penetration depends upon many factors but the general guide is that penetration varies inversely with frequency. A rough guide is that the useful image is around 100 wavelengths deep so for lower frequencies where the wavelength increases, the useful depth of field also increases.
  b. Aliasing of the pulsed Doppler signal can be eliminated by decreasing the scan depth.
     True: Aliasing occurs when the sample rate is insufficient to unambiguously determine the wave frequency. The sample frequency can be considered to be the same as the line refresh rate and so if this is increased then the frequency that it can be used to determine also increases. The line refresh rate can be increased by reducing the depth of field since the time taken for the echo to return is also reduced.
  c. Increasing the frequency only increases resolution in a harmonic image.
     False: US uses the physics of wave propagation to form the image. Huygen's principle is often used to consider how the wave front propagates, which is assumed to be a line of single point sources which combine to give the wavefront. One consequence of this is to reveal that the limiting resolution is a wavelength even when considering a linear wavefront and this is irrespective of the technique used.
  d. Turning on Doppler imaging will reduce the frame rate.
     True: Modern scanners have the capacity to process data very rapidly but if there are additional data to be derived from the returning echo, then additional time is required to process and display it. Even with complex parallel processing, there is likely to be a reduction in frame rate.
  e. Improving the image by the use of multiple focal zones has no effect on the frame rate.
     False: In order for focal zones to be formed it is necessary to reapply the delays onto the transducer. This does take time which will reduce the frame rate.

Q6.18 Basic physics

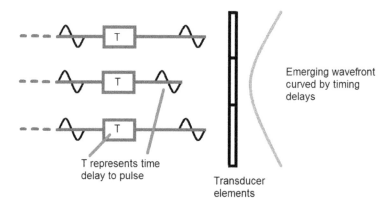

T represents time
delay to pulse

Transducer
elements

Emerging wavefront
curved by timing
delays

In phased arrays and mechanical sectors, the ability to focus and steer the US beam arises from the selective firing of individual transducer elements. The shape this gives to the propagating wave front depends upon the distribution of the delays and so the focus and steering can be controlled electronically without relying on mechanical constructions such as mechanical sectors, which are prone to wear, delay and also suffer from having a focus that is fixed.

Concerning modern transducers (true or false)
    a. A non-focused wave front requires a progression of delays across the transducer with equivalent delays between each element.
    b. Image quality can be improved by a process known as dynamic receive.
    c. The large number of elements in a phased array increases the focal region volume.
    d. Element sizes of around 1 mm are used in phased arrays.
    e. The phased array can be considered to be a single aperture.

Answers

a. A non-focused wave front requires a progression of delays across the transducer with equivalent delays between each element.

True: For a plane wave (non-focused) the wave will progress from each element in a given direction and the extent to which it travels with regard to the adjacent element will be constant along the transducer. Imagine a long line of individuals and each individual starts to run forward separated by 1 s from his neighbour. A line connecting the runners will be at an angle. This is a representation rather than exact analogy!

b. Image quality can be improved by a process known as dynamic receive.

True: This is the reverse of dynamic steering. Echoes returning from a boundary have further to go to the elements at the periphery of the probe and hence, under certain conditions, delays can be added to the time of the returning echoes to compensate for the additional return path.

c. The large number of elements in a phased array increases the focal region volume.

False: The large number of elements permits the focal volume to be much smaller as a result of improved destructive super-imposition of the waves.

d. Element sizes of around 1 mm are used in phased arrays.

False: The elements need to be smaller than a wavelength for them to be considered as point sources. US wavelengths are typically a few tenths of a millimetre or smaller.

e. The phased array can be considered to be a single aperture.

True: Because the elements are so small, they are considered to be point sources and hence together form a continuous transmitter.

Q6.19 Physics of ultrasound I

Aliasing is a term often associated with ultrasound and, in particular, spectral Doppler ultrasound, although mathematically it is a concept that can be applied to any technique that samples data and this includes magnetic resonance imaging and computed tomography. Aliasing can lead to the degradation of measured signals to such an extent that the spectral data cannot be used and hence its identification and management are important for the user. Most modern systems will identify when aliasing becomes likely but it remains important to be able to recognise aliasing and how its impact might be reduced or removed.

When managing aliasing (true or false)
    a. Aliasing in ultrasound is associated with blood flow velocities at the lower end of detectability.
    b. The Nyquist limit indicates the greatest flow velocity that can be unambiguously recorded.
    c. One option for eliminating aliasing is to reduce the image depth of field.
    d. Aliasing manifests itself on spectral Doppler ultrasound as inverted flow.
    e. Continuous wave Doppler ultrasound is not affected by aliasing.

Answers

a. Aliasing in ultrasound is associated with blood flow velocities at the lower end of detectability.

   False: Aliasing occurs where the sampling of the Doppler signal is insufficient to unambiguously identify its frequency. Hence this occurs at high blood velocities and is not related to a lower detectability.

b. The Nyquist limit indicates the greatest flow velocity that can be unambiguously recorded.

   True: The Nyquist limit is the highest frequency that can be unambiguously detected for a given sampling rate. Alternatively, it can be interpreted as the sample rate necessary to properly record a given shifted frequency.

c. One option for eliminating aliasing is to reduce the image depth of field.

   True: Reducing the depth of field decreases the transit time of the echoes and hence the pulse repetition frequency and sample rates also increase.

d. Aliasing manifests itself on spectral Doppler ultrasound as inverted flow.

   False: It usually manifests itself as reflected flow as in the diagram above. Inverted flow is flow that is opposing the flow being measured.

e. Continuous wave Doppler ultrasound is not affected by aliasing.

   True: Being continuous, the detected Doppler shift is also continuous but does require a dedicated transducer.

Q6.20 Physics of ultrasound II

One developing area in ultrasound imaging is transducer design. The design of the ultrasound transducer is not simply one of ergonomics. The design of the transducer goes a long way to maximising its use especially in small or confined spaces. This has been the case for some years now for transvaginal or transrectal scanning but transoesophogeal scanning is also now offered and consideration is being given to transluminal scanning although there remain difficulties in miniaturisation and also in how to meaningfully display the final images.

Considering the design of the transducer (true or false)
- a. Transoesophogeal transducers enable a higher frame rate image of cardiac structures.
- b. A single broken transducer element is unlikely to seriously reduce the efficacy of the ultrasound image.
- c. The edge elements of transducers can be fired so as to minimise side-lobe artefacts.
- d. The matching layer permits the more efficient transmission of ultrasound into the patient.
- e. Curvilinear probes are used where there is a need for small footprints.

Answers

a. Transoesophogeal transducers enable a higher frame rate image of cardiac structures.

   True: the transducer in question can be located much closer to the heart than if performed extra-corporeally. This reduces the echo transit time and hence the frame rate can be much higher.

b. A single broken transducer element is unlikely to seriously reduce the efficacy of the ultrasound image.

   True: A single broken element will have an effect very superficially, but can be compensated for by the large number of remaining transducer elements. However, where superficial scanning is important, then corrective action may be necessary. A missing element may suggest other faults so is often checked and corrected for.

c. The edge elements of transducers can be fired so as to minimise side-lobe artefacts.

   True: This is a technique known as apodisation and is a diffraction and interference effect that can cause artefacts. The timing of the edge elements are altered to partially cancel the waves which contribute to the side lobes.

d. The matching layer permits the more efficient transmission of ultrasound into the patient.

   True: the matching layer helps in reducing the acoustic impedance step between soft tissue and the transducer which would otherwise lead to almost total reflection from the boundary.

e. Curvilinear probes are used where there is a need for small footprints.

   False: Curvilinear probes tend to be large in comparison to phased arrays and hence have a large footprint. This is useful for imaging when a wide field of view is helpful at shallow depths.

Q6.21 Ultrasound

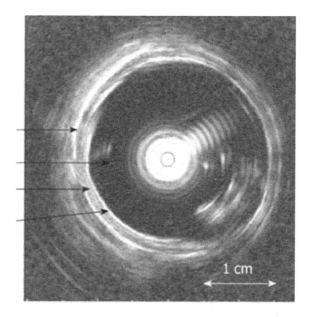

Ultrasound is considered to be very safe although there is a growing concern about where the thresholds of risk lie especially in relation to heating and cavitation. Furthermore, the ultrasound image is complex to interpret and expensive training is necessary, in particular for complex anatomy or difficult conditions.

Some limitations of use with ultrasound (true or false)

    a. Ultrasound is contra-indicated where vascularity is compromised, thus reducing heat dissipation.

    b. A typical pulse length comprises around three wavelengths.

    c. The type of tissue can be inferred from its appearance in the ultrasound image.

    d. Harmonic imaging increases contrast but decreases resolution.

    e. Tissue Harmonic Imaging is most marked at shallow penetration.

Answers

a. Ultrasound is contra-indicated where vascularity is compromised, thus reducing heat dissipation.

False: Ultrasound can be very useful in investigating blood perfusion, although care has to be taken where there might be an infection risk since contact has to be made with the area under investigation.

b. A typical pulse length comprises around three wavelengths.

True: Ideally one wavelength would be used since that would be the best possible resolution, but the creation of the pulse means that a practical limit is around three wavelengths.

c. The type of tissue can be inferred from its appearance in the ultrasound image.

False: Tissue characterisation is not possible using current techniques. What is usually meant is that the location and shape can be used to determine the tissue under investigation.

d. Harmonic imaging increases contrast but decreases resolution.

False: Harmonic imaging takes advantage of higher frequencies generated in the returning echo. This is associated with higher resolution. It is also often associated with higher contrast, although this depends upon the depth of the image.

e. Tissue Harmonic Imaging is most marked at shallow penetration.

False: THI requires a relatively large transit distance for the required harmonics to develop.

Q6.22 Safety in ultrasound

How the patient responds to the risk from ultrasound can vary. Some patients report that they can hear the ultrasound, but it is unclear how this can occur since the penetration of ultrasound at diagnostic frequencies is very short. What is clear though, is that ultrasound is a form of energy and as such can interact with tissue by a variety of mechanisms and those of most interest at diagnostic levels are heating and tissue disruption by cavitation.

When considering the safety of patients and staff in ultrasound (true or false)
   a. There is a risk to the patient's hearing from the excessive use of diagnostic ultrasound.
   b. Thermal index is of more relevance to the patient than mechanical index.
   c. The introduction of contrast agents increases the risk from cavitation.
   d. The risk from cavitation increases inversely with frequency.
   e. Thermal damage is often found in patients having undergone extended ultrasound procedures.

Answers

a. There is a risk to the patient's hearing from the excessive use of diagnostic ultrasound.

   False: Ultrasound frequencies do not propagate through air and in any case the ultrasound has a frequency that is well in excess of the upper hearing threshold. What some patients hear is the electronic noise from the transducer.

b. Thermal index is of more relevance to the patient than mechanical index.

   True: The major concern is from tissue heating although in some circumstances, the risk from cavitation can be of concern, especially where contrast agents are used.

c. The introduction of contrast agents increases the risk from cavitation.

   True: The small encapsulated bubbles can collapse during insonation, especially at high intensities, which leads to localised tissue damage.

d. The risk from cavitation increases inversely with frequency.

   False: The relationship is complex but it is the inverse of the square root of frequency.

e. Thermal damage is often found in patients having undergone extended ultrasound procedures.

   False: Thermal damage is not routinely found at all.

IOP Publishing

Scientific Basis of the Royal College of Radiologists Fellowship (2nd Edition)

Illustrated questions and answers

Malcolm Sperrin and John Winder

Chapter 7

Magnetic resonance imaging

MRI is a highly complex modality that utilises physics that is far from intuitive. The design and manufacture of the systems is also extremely complex and this may make MRI a daunting prospect for study. However, a comprehensive understanding of MRI is often beyond the bounds of many medical physicists and there is no requirement for the radiology trainee to have a detailed knowledge of the underpinning science. The techniques can be understood by a familiarity with some generic concepts and an acceptance of some esoteric aspects. Safety is important and there is a need for a knowledge of key exposure limits and also the nature of some of the hazards. MRI is also a useful technique in that it is non-ionizing in nature but known hazards do still exist and are present for patients and staff alike. MRI has the benefit of being able to generate different image contrast by exploiting different tissue properties which enhance the diagnostic tools available to the radiologist.

Q7.1 The source of the magnetic resonance signal

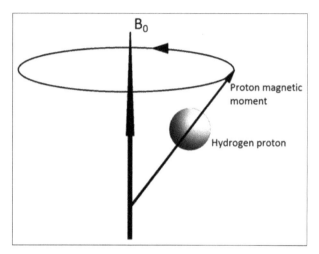

The vertical black arrow in the figure represents the direction of the main magnetic field (B_0) generated by the MR scanner. For a 1.5 T or 3.0 T 'tunnel' magnet this magnetic field is horizontal through the bore of the magnet. The proton (nucleus of the hydrogen atom) generates a small magnetic field of its own, called the proton magnetic moment and, in the presence of B_0, precesses around the main magnetic field tracing the path indicated by the circle. The rate or frequency of precession is defined by the Larmor equation (64 MHz at 1.5 T). The frequency is dependent on the main magnetic field strength and a constant for the proton (gyromagnetic ratio),

$$\text{Larmor frequency} = \gamma \cdot B_0$$

where γ = gyromagnetic frequency and B_0 is the strength of the magnetic field.

When detecting the MR signal, we actually measure the net (total) effect of all proton magnetic moments within a given volume (voxel). This total is called the net magnetic moment (M_0). It is made up of the difference between protons lying parallel and anti-parallel to the external magnetic field (these two states are referred to as different spin states).

Concerning the MR signal (true or false)
   a. The MR signal can be detected because there are equal numbers of protons in two different energy states.
   b. An external magnetic field causes proton magnetic moments to precess.
   c. Precession of the proton magnetic moment produces a motion like a spinning top.
   d. Many proton magnetic moments generate a net magnetic moment (M_0).
   e. Proton magnetic moments always point in the same direction as the external magnetic field.

Answers

a. The MR signal can be detected because there are equal numbers of protons in two different energy states.

False: There are two different energy states, one where the proton magnetic moment is aligned with the magnetic field and one where the moment is in opposition to the main field. The net magnetic moment is due to the difference in the number of protons in each of these energy states.

b. An external magnetic field causes proton magnetic moments to precess.

True: Using the Larmor equation, if there was no magnetic field present then B_0 would be zero and the Larmor frequency would be zero (apart from the presence of the Earth's magnetic field) and therefore there would be no precessional motion.

c. Precession of the proton magnetic moment produces a motion like a spinning top.

True: A rapidly rotating spinning top does not precess but spins around its own axis, however, as it slows, its motion is precession.

d. Many proton magnetic moments generate a net magnetic moment (M_0).

True: The net magnetic moment is so called as it is the vector sum of all the individual proton magnetic moments within a sample.

e. Proton magnetic moments always point in the same direction as the external magnetic field.

False: As described in answer a, there are two energy states which may be defined by their alignment or opposition to an externally applied magnetic field.

Q7.2 Magnetic resonance signal: the net magnetic moment

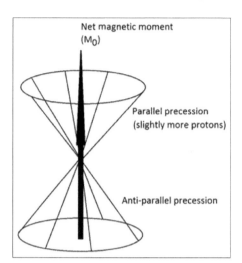

If we consider a small portion of tissue, like a cubic millimetre of fat, then all the hydrogen protons in the voxel of fat, when subjected to a large external magnetic field, will either align themselves in parallel ('spin up') to the external field (B_0) or anti-parallel ('spin down'). The impact of protons arranging themselves like this is that their individual magnetic moments cancel each other out (as they are the same magnitude but pointing in opposing directions). Note they are precessing around at the Larmor frequency and therefore this is an average or net effect.

There is a greater number of protons lying parallel with the magnetic field, therefore there is a net magnetic moment generated by the protons in the same direction as the external magnetic field. It is this excess magnetic moment that is detected using our patient RF coils. Generally, the greater the net magnetic moment (M_0) the greater the MR signal (also referred to as proton density).

Concerning the net magnetic moment (true or false)
    a. The net magnetic moment can be detected because there are equal numbers of protons in two different energy states.
    b. An external magnetic field forces protons to exist on one of two energy states.
    c. There are a greater number of protons parallel to B_0 than antiparallel.
    d. The net magnetic moment is related to the proton density of the tissue.
    e. The net magnetization is the vector sum of all protons in the voxel.

Answers

   a. The net magnetic moment can be detected because there are equal numbers of protons in two different energy states.

      False: Although the are two populations of protons in different energy states, the reason the net magnetization can be detected is because it is rotating in a plane that enables an electric current to be induced in a coil.

   b. An external magnetic field forces protons to exist on one of two energy states.

      True: The energy states are referred to as parallel or anti-parallel and there is a slightly greater population of protons that exist in the anti-parallel condition. It is these excess protons that give rise to the MR signal.

   c. There are a greater number of protons parallel to B_0 than anti-parallel.

      False: It is the other way around, more protons are anti-parallel.

   d. The net magnetic moment is related to the proton density of the tissue.

      True: The proton density is the concentration of mobile hydrogen within tissues and one of the main determinants of the MR signal.

   e. The net magnetization is the vector sum of all protons in the voxel.

      True: In many circumstances throughout the generation of the MR signal, individual proton magnetic moments may be pointing in differing directions, therefore the net effect is a vector sum of all these.

Q7.3 Magnetic resonance image contrast (image weighting)

(a) Proton density   (b) T1   (c) T2

MR is very flexible as an imaging system in that it can acquire images with a variety of image contrasts. Shown in the figure are three transverse images of the brain, illustrating a) proton density, b) longitudinal relaxation (T1) and c) transverse relaxation (T2) weighted image contrast. This means the MR signal strength within the image is dependent on the tissue values for each of these parameters. These image contrasts are based on different tissue MR properties. The simplest to understand is proton density weighting—it is called weighting because the signals are based on the proton density of each tissue. In this case a tissue with higher proton density will be brighter in the image and a tissue with low proton density (lack of water content in bone, for example) will be darker as it has generated a lower signal.

Concerning MR image contrast (true or false)
   a. Proton density differences between soft tissues are around 50%.
   b. An external magnetic field causes proton magnetic moments to precess.
   c. The Larmor frequency is inversely related to the main magnetic field strength.
   d. The free induction decay signal occurs due to relaxation processes.
   e. T2 relaxation occurs after T1 relaxation has completed.

Answers

    a. Proton density differences between soft tissues are around 50%.
        False: The variation in proton density in soft tissues is much less at around 10%, which results in images of limited contrast.

    b. An external magnetic field causes proton magnetic moments to precess.
        True: The proton magnetic moments interact with a magnetic field which causes them to wobble or to precess around the magnetic field.

    c. The Larmor frequency is inversely related to the main magnetic field strength.
        False: As the equation demonstrates, the Larmor frequency is directly related to the magnetic field strength.

    d. The free induction decay signal occurs due to relaxation processes.
        True: Free induction decay is a description of the MR signal as it falls off due to the relaxation processes.

    e. T2 relaxation occurs after T1 relaxation has completed.
        False: Both relaxation processes begin as soon as the RF is switched off and generally the T2 relaxation will have completed before the T1 relaxation.

Q7.4 Transverse magnetization

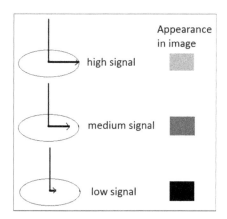

A 90° RF pulse is used in MR pulse sequences to create transverse magnetization. The absorption of the RF energy causes the net magnetic moment (M_0) to tip out of alignment with the main magnetic field (B_0). It contains enough power to make M_0 precess in the transverse plane. The 90° RF pulse gathers all the protons together and causes them to precess in unison (coherently or in phase). It is essential to create transverse magnetization as this can be detected, whereas non-transverse magnetization cannot. This is the only 'configuration' of magnetization that will induce an electric current into the patient RF coil. As the net magnetization precesses in the transverse plane it generates a signal that is oscillating at the Larmor frequency.

Transverse magnetization (true or false)
  a. Is always measured in MR.
  b. Is created using a 90° RF pulse a spin echo pulse sequence.
  c. Decays at a rate governed by a combination of T1 and T2.
  d. Lies in the same direction as the main magnetic field B_0.
  e. Oscillates at 64 MHz at 1.5 T.

Answers

a. Is always measured in MR.

True: Transverse magnetization is created in MR so that the motion of the magnetic vector is such that it can induce an electric current into a loop or coil.

b. Is created using a 90° RF pulse in a spin echo pulse sequence.

True: The 90° RF pulse tips the net magnetic moment out of alignment with the main magnetic field into the transverse plane so that it can be detected.

c. Decays at a rate governed by a combination of T1 and T2.

True: Both relaxation processes simultaneously cause a reduction in the net transverse magnetic moment.

d. Lies in the same direction as the main magnetic field B_0.

False: The transverse magnetization lies at 90° to the main field.

e. Oscillates at 64 MHz at 1.5 T.

True: The transverse magnetization rotates around the main magnetic field at the Larmor frequency.

Q7.5 Metal artefacts in magnetic resonance imaging

Aneurysm clip   Hip implant   Knee reconstruction

Metal artefacts are common in MR and are a subset of susceptibility artefacts. Susceptibility is the ability of a material to take up a magnetic field to which it is temporarily exposed. In the case of metal (ferromagnetic materials such as iron, cobalt or nickel) the homogeneity of the main magnetic field is disturbed by the magnetic field generated in the metal. This is demonstrated in the examples above. The homogeneity of the main field may be locally disturbed and characteristic no signal adjacent to high signal areas are observed in the image. More subtle effects of susceptibility may occur near tissue–air interfaces and produce unusual signals that may be misinterpreted as pathology. The main methods for reducing the effects of susceptibility are to reduce voxel size, reduce echo time (TE) time and use spin echo rather than gradient echo sequences. Other common artefacts like movement or flow are dependent on the phase encoding direction, that is, they appear to propagate along this direction. Chemical artefacts such as chemical shift or signal cancellation due to phase interaction of water and fat signals occur in the frequency encoding direction.

Artefacts on MR due to metal implants are (true or false)
  a. Greater at higher field strength.
  b. Worse on spin echo images than gradient echo images.
  c. Independent of the read and phase encoding directions.
  d. Greater at shorter TEs.
  e. Reduced by frequency selective fat suppression.

Answers

a. Greater at higher field strength.

True: The magnetic susceptibility of a material, metal in this case, is directly dependent on the magnetic field it is immersed in and increases as the field strength increases.

b. Worse on spin echo images than gradient echo images.

False: The 180° RF refocusing pulse in a spin echo sequence reduces the impact of proton dephasing due to magnetic field inhomogeneities. However, the gradient echo sequence uses magnetic field gradients to refocus the dephasing protons which do not reduce the impact of magnetic field inhomogeneities.

c. Independent of the read and phase encoding directions.

True: Susceptibility affects the magnetic field homogeneity in all directions.

d. Greater at shorter TEs.

False: Shorter TEs do not have an impact on the degree of metal artefacts.

e. Reduced by frequency selective fat suppression.

False: Frequency selective fat suppression uses a narrow band RF pulse to excite fat protons only and has no impact on metal artefacts.

Q7.6 The spin echo pulse sequence

The spin echo pulse sequence is so called as it creates a signal (called the 'echo'), from the protons (spins) that are present in the tissue. It uses a 90° RF pulse to create transverse magnetization. After this RF pulse is switched off (of the order of milliseconds), the protons begin to dephase and their magnetizations become out of alignment with each other (this has the effect of reducing the strength of transverse magnetization that the patient RF coil would detect). It is at this point that a 180° RF pulse is transmitted into the patient to reverse the dephasing effect and the proton magnetizations become re-aligned to create the signal (an echo). The signal is read at a time called the TE. In a spin echo pulse sequence, the body relaxes after the RF pulse for a period of time called the repetition time (TR). TR and TE are used to control contrast. Typical TR and TE times are given in the table below.

Image weighting	TR (ms)	TE (ms)
Proton density	Long (2000–4000)	Short (10–20)
T1	Short (400–700)	Short (10–20)
T2	Long (2000–4000)	Long (80–120)

The spin echo pulse sequence (true or false)
   a. Can generate proton density, T1 and T2 weighted images.
   b. Produces images that suffer from magnetic field inhomogeneity.
   c. Creates the MR signal (the echo) using a 90° RF pulse.
   d. Uses the RF sequence 90–180°....90–180° repeatedly separated by TE.
   e. Is programmed to have a TR of between 400 and 700 ms to obtain a T2 weighted image.

Answers

a. Can generate proton density, T1 and T2 weighted images.

   True: The spin echo pulse sequence is very versatile and can generate these image weights using different TR and TE settings.

b. Produces images that suffer from magnetic field inhomogeneity.

   False: The spin echo pulse sequence uses a 180° refocusing RF pulse which reduces the impact of magnetic field inhomogeneity by reversing the dephasing caused by imperfections in the main magnetic field.

c. Creates the MR signal (the echo) using a 90° RF pulse.

   False: This question is slightly ambiguous as the 90° RF pulse is used to create transverse magnetization, however, it is the 180° RF pulse that refocuses the dephasing protons which come together to produce the signal.

d. Uses the RF sequence 90–180°....90–180° repeatedly separated by TE.

   False: The spin echo pulse sequence does use this combination of RF pulses, however, they are separated by the TR.

e. Is programmed to have a TR of between 400 and 700 ms to obtain a T2 weighted image.

   False: As from the table you will see that the TR required to generate T2 weighted images is at least 2000 ms.

Q7.7 Magnetic resonance safety: main magnetic field

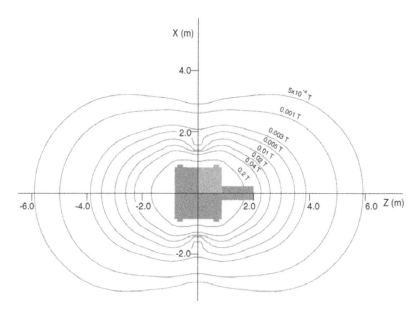

The main hazards associated with MRI are the main magnetic field, the RF pulses, the oscillating magnetic field gradients, acoustic noise and the presence of a cryogen. Ferromagnetic materials attracted by the magnetic field will contain significant amounts of iron, nickel or cobalt. A superconducting magnet is always on. An area around the scanner defined by the 3 mT contour is defined as the inner controlled zone and generally the magnet room contains the 5 mT contour.

Concerning MR safety (true or false)
   a. Access to the MR controlled area requires people to be fully screened.
   b. The fringe field is close the MR machine.
   c. Some UK and European coins are magnetic as they contain cobalt.
   d. MR compatible means that the object is safe to bring into the magnet room.
   e. The inner zone is defined by a 300 mT contour.

Answers

   a. Access to the MR controlled area requires people to be fully screened.

      True: The controlled area may enable people to be exposed to a field strength of 0.5 mT or greater and this may be hazardous to people with certain types of implant.

   b. The fringe field is close the MR machine.

      False: The fringe field is the weak magnetic field that exists well away from the scanner and its extent will depend on the main magnet field strength and the presence of shielding.

   c. Some UK and European coins are magnetic as they contain cobalt.

      False: Some coins are magnetic but it is due to their nickel content.

   d. MR compatible means that the object is safe to bring into the magnet room.

      False: If something is deemed MR compatible it may be safe to use in certain conditions but not all. An electronic device may function well within the magnet room but fail as it is brought close to the strong magnetic field, therefore it is compatible for a specific condition.

   e. The inner zone is defined by a 300 mT contour.

      False: The inner zone in a MR unit is defined by the 3 mT contour.

Q7.8 Magnetic resonance imaging parameters

The signal used to create an MR image is dependent on many factors including the proton density of the tissue, the imaging parameters during acquisition, type of equipment used and presence of a contrast agent. We wish to achieve a SNR suitable for creating a diagnostic image. Imaging factors, such as slice width, pixel size, RF receiver bandwidth, the number of excitations (NEX), TR and TE, influence the SNR. Lower resolution is associated with greater signal, narrower bandwidth results in reduced noise, therefore increased SNR; the SNR will increase with increasing NEX. Increasing TR and decreasing TE will result in increased signal.

Concerning MRI parameters (true or false)
  a. Increase in SNR is directly related to increasing NEX.
  b. A large voxel will produce a better SNR than a small voxel.
  c. Thin slices decrease spatial resolution.
  d. Changing the bandwidth from 32 kHz to 16 kHz can affect image noise.
  e. Changing the image matrix from 256 to 512 will decrease the SNR for the same imaging conditions.

Answers

a. Increase in SNR is directly related to increasing NEX.

True: Increasing the NEX is the same as increasing the number of individual signals for a given slice and averaging them together. Averaging signals has the effect of reducing noise as it cancels out, whilst the signal is built upon.

b. A large voxel will produce a better SNR than a small voxel.

True: The signal is directly proportional to the voxel size so any increase in the voxel dimension means that more protons are available to contribute to the net magnetic moment.

c. Thin slices decrease spatial resolution.

False: The spatial resolution of an MR system is governed by the pixel size (image matrix and FOV) and the slice thickness. A thinner slice, 2 mm compared to 5 mm, will enable the scanner to resolve smaller objects as they will be less obscured by the partial volume effect.

d. Changing the bandwidth from 32 kHz to 16 kHz can affect image noise.

True: As the bandwidth has decreased by a factor of two, the scanner will collect a lot less noise with the signal and therefore there will be a direct impact on the SNR.

e. Changing the image matrix from 256 to 512 will decrease the SNR for the same imaging conditions.

True: Changing the matrix size described will quadruple the number of pixels in a given FOV and therefore their area will be reduced by a factor of four. This has a direct impact on voxel volume and therefore on signal.

Q7.9 Magnetic resonance technology

A superconducting MR magnet has its niobium–titanium alloy coil cooled by liquid helium to 4 K (−269 °C). This coil is a single wire that is many kilometres long and carries hundreds of amps of electric current to produce the main magnetic field. A secondary set of coils within the main magnet, called shim coils, produce magnetic fields that make small adjustments to the main field and increase its homogeneity. The RF patient RF coils are used to transmit and receive RF EM radiation in the MHz region (around 64 MHz at 1.5 T). The magnet room is kept 'RF quiet' using a copper box build within the walls of the room and is called the Faraday cage.

Concerning MR technology
    a. Shim coils are used to reduce the fringe field outside the magnet room.
    b. The RF cabin prevents contamination of the MR signal from external RF sources.
    c. Multi-element RF patient coils can be used to improve the image SNR.
    d. The coolant in an MR scanner is at 400 K.
    e. The main magnetic field inhomogeneity should be around one in a thousand.

Answers

a. Shim coils are used to reduce the fringe field outside the magnet room.

   False: Shim coils are used to homogenize the main magnetic field to vary only a few parts per million over 30–40 cm for imaging. The reduction in fringe field is achieved using active coils or counter coils which generate magnetic fields to constrain the main field.

b. The RF cabin prevents contamination of the MR signal from external RF sources.

   True: The RF cabin, also called the Faraday cage, is a complete copper box built within the walls of the MR examination room. It prevents potentially contaminating RF radiation from entering the room.

c. Multi-element RF patient coils can be used to improve the image SNR.

   True: These RF coils are also referred as phased array coils, where the RF detection is performed using multiple receiving coils within one unit. This brings the individual coils closer to the MR signal therefore increasing SNR.

d. The coolant in an MR scanner is at 400 K.

   False: The liquid helium is at 4 K ($-269\,°C$).

e. The main magnetic field inhomogeneity should be around one in a thousand.

   False: The main magnetic field homogeneity is required to be a few parts per million (variation in field strength of a few microTesla) over the imaging volume and even higher than this for spectroscopic examinations.

Q7.10 Gradient magnetic fields

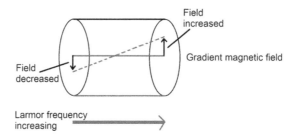

Gradient magnetic fields are produced within the main magnet housing by a special set of coils and enable small linear changes to be made to the strength of the main magnetic field. They are switched on and off rapidly during image acquisition and produce a loud noise as the coil vibrates within its housing. These changes to the main magnetic field cause changes in the Larmor frequency of the protons across the body and enable spatial localization of the MR signal. Gradient fields are also used in gradient echo imaging to generate the MR echo (signal) and to remove (spoil) transverse magnetization.

Gradient magnetic fields (true or false)
   a. Generate electrical currents within the patient.
   b. Are time varying and are used to spatially localize the MR signal.
   c. Are of the order of 30 T per metre in a typical 1.5 T system.
   d. Can be used to refocus the MR signal in gradient echo sequences.
   e. Produce sound levels of around 90–100 dBA.

Answers

a. Generate electrical currents within the patient.

True: A time varying magnetic field (the gradient magnetic fields) generates and electric field, which in turn causes electrical current to flow in the body as it is a conductor (it has ions flowing through it). For very fast gradients these currents have the potential to stimulate nerves, resulting in uncontrolled muscle movements.

b. Are time varying and are used to spatially localize the MR signal.

True: Gradient magnetic fields are switched on and off rapidly and are used to provide frequency encoding and phase encoding within a slice to determine where the MR signal is coming from and also to spatially localize individual slices.

c. Are of the order of 30 T per metre in a typical 1.5 T system.

False: Gradients are typically measured in milliTesla per metre ($mT\ m^{-1}$) so this figure is out by a large amount. The figure is sometimes confused with the manufacturer specification of gradient performance using the rise time. This is measured in Tesla per metre per second ($T\ m^{-1}\ s^{-1}$). Therefore a system's gradients may be defined as having a strength of $33\ mT\ m^{-1}$ with a rise time of $125\ T\ m^{-1}\ s^{-1}$.

d. Can be used to refocus the MR signal in gradient echo sequences.

True: If a gradient is switched on, protons within a voxel will precess at different Larmor frequencies and cause them to dephase or become out of alignment. If the gradient is subsequently reversed then the voxels will rephase due to experiencing a new Larmor frequency and eventually come into alignment with each other forming an MR signal (echo).

e. Produce sound levels of around 90–100 dBA.

True: The gradient coils are energized with large electrical currents which are switched on and off rapidly. This results in the coils vibrating within the housing and causing high noise levels.

Q7.11 Relaxation times in magnetic resonance imaging

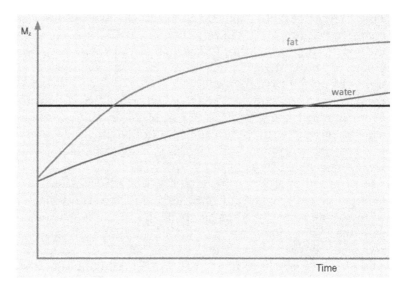

During MRI, the patient (their protons) is exposed to RF EM radiation at a proton's Larmor frequency (~64 MHz at 1.5 T). Protons absorb this energy. As soon as the RF pulse is turned off, the protons immediately begin to lose this energy by two processes, T1 and T2 relaxation. Within the body, these relaxation processes are defined by the times at which each tissue loses energy. The relaxation times, T1 and T2, are measured in milliseconds and vary widely throughout the body by tissue type. T1 relaxation is also referred to as spin–lattice relaxation as protons (spins) are continuously on the move by thermal agitation of the surrounding molecules. T2 relaxation is referred to as spin–spin relaxation as there is interaction by tiny local magnetic fields generated by individual protons close to each other. In some cases the local magnetic field is increased due to the presence of other protons and therefore the Larmor frequency is increased. Close by, the local magnetic field may be reduced by proton interaction and the Larmor frequency is reduced. The overall effect is dephasing and signal loss.

Concerning relaxation times in MRI (true or false)
   a. Magnetic field inhomogeneity affects T1 more than T2.
   b. T1 contrast in gradient echo images depends on the flip angle.
   c. Gadolinium based contrast agents have more effect on T2 than T1.
   d. The T1 relaxation time of fat is relatively long.
   e. Tissues with short T2 relaxation times have low signal in T2 weighted images.

Answers

a. Magnetic field inhomogeneity affects T1 more than T2.

   False: T1 relaxation is the return of the net magnetic moment to the resting position precessing around the main magnetic field axis and therefore is unaffected by magnetic field inhomogeneties. T1 is dependent on the overall scanner field strength, lengthening with increasing magnetic field. T2 is the component of increased relaxation due to magnetic field inhomgeneities.

b. T1 contrast in gradient echo images depends on the flip angle.

   True: Gradient echo images use a short TR and TE to produce T1 weighting and the degree of weighting is controlled by the flip angle of the excitation RF pulse.

c. Gadolinium based contrast agents have more effect on T2 than T1.

   False: Normal dose gadolinium has a marked impact on the T1 relaxation time of tissues causing them to reduce significantly. However, at higher doses a T2 effect may be observed where there is signal loss.

d. The T1 relaxation time of fat is relatively long.

   False: The T1 of fat is around 250 ms at 1.0 T which is significantly shorter than many other tissues. Fat therefore appears bright on a T1 weighted image.

e. Tissues with short T2 relaxation times have low signal in T2 weighted images.

   True: The MR signal from a tissue with a short relaxation time (for example, liver or muscle), will be low as the signal will decay rapidly. Remember, 99% of the MR signal will have decayed by five times the tissue T2.

Q7.12 Fast/turbo spin echo magnetic resonance imaging

Echo train (ETL = 4)

In conventional spin echo imaging the protons are excited by a 90° RF pulse; the size of the MR signal (echo) is measured after a 180° RF pulse is applied. The body is then allowed to relax for a period called TR. The process is repeated for the number of phase encoding steps required to build up the image matrix. For fast spin echo imaging, multiple 180° RF pulses are applied in quick succession and an MR signal (new echo) is measured after each pulse. This is carried out a specific number of times called the echo train length (ETL) and may be 4, 8, 16 or even longer. Fast imaging has the effect of reducing the scan time and the longer the ETL the shorter the scan time.

Concerning fast spin echo imaging (true or false)
   a. One phase encode step is acquired per excitation.
   b. Increasing the number of echoes results in a greater average TE.
   c. Specific absorption rates (SARs) are higher compared to echo planar imaging.
   d. Fast spin echo imaging is often used for T2 weighted imaging.
   e. Fast spin echo imaging is faster than conventional spin echo imaging.

Answers

a. One phase encode step is acquired per excitation.

False: If multiple 180° RF pulses are applied then a new phase encoding step is collected for each pulse. Therefore, multiple phase encoding steps are collected for each 90° RF excitation, subsequently reducing the NEX.

b. Increasing the number of echoes results in a greater average TE.

True: For a longer ETL with the same echo spacing, the average TE for the overall sequence will be increased.

c. SARs are higher compared to echo planar imaging.

True: Echo planar imaging uses one 90° RF pulse followed by a sequence of gradients to refocus the MR signal. The fast spin echo sequence uses multiple 180° RF pulses and therefore more RF is delivered to the patient increasing the SAR.

d. Fast spin echo imaging is often used for T2 weighted imaging.

True: There is inherently more T2 weighting in fast spin echo sequences as echoes are collected at longer average TEs. More recently, with the advent of faster gradients and RF technology, the average TE can be reduced along with limited ETL to produce T1 weighted images with little T2 weighting present.

e. Fast spin echo imaging is faster than conventional spin echo imaging.

True: As the name suggests, the fast or turbo action of having an increased ETL will result in collecting more phase encoding gradients per excitation and therefore reduce overall imaging time (even though fewer slices can be collected per TR).

Q7.13 Fat suppression techniques

There are many reasons why suppressing signal from fat within the body is useful in MR. Fat saturation by selective excitation uses an RF pulse tuned to the fat protons only (they differ from water protons by 220 Hz at 1.5 T) so that they are 'saturated' at the beginning of any pulse sequence. When the rest of the sequence is performed only water protons respond. This technique depends on good magnetic field homogeneity and is best over small FOV. Specific pulse sequences (the STIR and Dixon techniques) may be used where the timing of the sequence ensures that very low or zero signal is obtained from fat. The Dixon technique is especially effective as it uses carefully chosen TEs where the fat/water protons are in phase and out of phase with each other. It works well in areas of high susceptibility where other techniques do not perform well.

Concerning fat suppression (true or false)
  a. STIR images require good static field homogeneity.
  b. Frequency selective fat suppression is useful with a gadolinium based contrast agent.
  c. In phase and out of phase images are acquired at the same TE.
  d. Fat and water may be excited separately.
  e. Frequency selective fat suppression is better with larger FOV.

Answers

a. STIR images require good static field homogeneity.

   False: Both fat and water protons are excited in this sequence and the reduction in fat signal is achieved by introducing an inversion pulse where the fat signal is removed and all other tissues are unaffected.

b. Frequency selective fat suppression is useful with a gadolinium based contrast agent.

   True: Changes in T1 to tissues by the presence of gadolinium may cause the tissues to have a T1 similar to fat and therefore suffer from suppression when not desired. A frequency selective technique would not have the impact on the contrast agent.

c. In phase and out of phase images are acquired at the same TE.

   False: After excitation by the 90° RF pulse, both fat and water protons quickly become out of phase with each other and by 2.3 ms they are actually spinning around in directions in opposition to each other and then at 4.6 ms they are in phase again. Signals recorded at out of phase and in phase TEs are used to separate the fat and water signals.

d. Fat and water may be excited separately.

   True: Fat protons and water protons have Larmor frequencies that differ by around 220 Hz at 1.5 T and therefore by using narrow band RF pulses either the fat or water protons can be made to resonate and preferentially absorb the RF.

e. Frequency selective fat suppression is better with larger FOV.

   False: A greater FOV may result in larger main magnetic field inhomogeneity (this is also compounded as the body distorts the magnetic field). To minimize the amount of variation in the fat proton Larmor frequency, the area of coverage (FOV) should be minimized.

Q7.14 Radio frequency safety

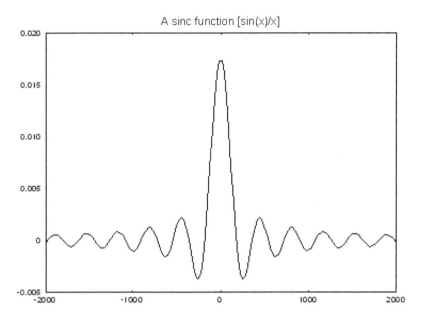

The RF waves used in MR are in the MHz range and are absorbed within the body. They may cause heating and also create a risk where metal or cables are present within the bore of the magnet. It is generally accepted that a rise of 1 °C may be tolerated by healthy people, however, temperature rise within the body is due to many factors, including clothing, air flow, ambient temperature and humidity. The limit to RF power delivered to the patient is governed by the SAR and is measured in W kg^{-1}.

Concerning RF safety (true or false)
    a. The main hazard from RF is nerve stimulation.
    b. Localized RF energy deposition to the limbs is the same as for the head.
    c. The patient is always weighed before scanning to ensure that the correct SAR is calculated.
    d. Tissues with low blood supply are sensitive to RF heating.
    e. A SAR of 4 W kg^{-1} applies to whole body RF exposure.

Answers

a. The main hazard from RF is nerve stimulation.

   False: The main hazard from RF EM radiation is from heating.

b. Localized RF energy deposition to the limbs is the same as for the head.

   False: There are fewer sensitive tissues within the limbs and heat is dissipated by blood vessel dilation if needed, therefore the SAR limit for limbs is higher than that for the head.

c. The patient is always weighed before scanning to ensure that the correct SAR is calculated.

   True: The patient's weight is added to the system when entering patient details and the SAR is calculated for their weight. If the SAR is exceeded, for example due to number of slices, the operator will be alerted to make changes before scanning can commence.

d. Tissues with low blood supply are sensitive to RF heating.

   True: The testes and the lens of the eye are susceptible due to their limited blood supply.

e. A SAR of $4\,\mathrm{W\,kg^{-1}}$ applies to whole body RF exposure.

   False: The SAR limit is $0.4\,\mathrm{W\,kg^{-1}}$ averaged over the whole body and is higher for head/torso and limbs.

Q7.15 Magnetic resonance image artefacts

MRI has a variety of artefacts associated with it, some of which are obvious. Others are very subtle and may confuse the clinical region of interest. Knowledge of the origin, appearance and management of artefacts is essential to avoid errors in decision making and to maximize the diagnostic potential.

Concerning MRI artefacts (true or false)
- a. Chemical shift occurs in the same direction as the flow artefact.
- b. The flow artefact occurs along the frequency encoding direction.
- c. The movement artefact occurs along the phase encoding direction.
- d. Metal artefacts are a form of susceptibility artefact.
- e. The phase encoding gradient is usually made across the length of the body to prevent wrap.

Answers

a. Chemical shift occurs in the same direction as the flow artefact.

False: The chemical shift arises as a result of partial screening of the magnetic field by fat molecules and hence the artefact occurs in the frequency direction. The flow artefact occurs because the volume that receives an excitation pulse is in a different position to the read-out pulse and hence is largely governed by the direction of flow.

b. The flow artefact occurs along the frequency encoding direction.

False: The flow artefact, which can appear as partial occlusion of the vessel in spin echo, is governed largely by the direction of flow of the blood and is not uniquely associated with a given encoding direction.

c. The movement artefact occurs along the phase encoding direction.

True: The movement artefact occurs largely in the phase encoding direction because an image is formed during each phase encoding cycle. The frequency encoding can be considered to be fixed and movement gives rise to blurring of boundaries or, if the movement is similar to the TR value, then ghosting can occur.

d. Metal artefacts are a form of susceptibility artefact.

True: Susceptibility is a term given where the local magnetic field is susceptible to corruption. This is usually as a result of embedded metal but can also arise from eddy currents in implants or even magnetic field disturbances from dental implants, makeup, etc.

e. The phase encoding gradient is usually made across the length of the body to prevent wrap.

False: Phase and frequency encoding are applied arbitrarily and can be swapped to reduce some types of artefact. If a feature is suspected to be an artefact, then swapping the direction of the encoding directions can cause the artefact to move or change appearance and is therefore useful in separating out anatomy from artefact.

Q7.16 Magnetic resonance safety I

MR safety is an important aspect of managing a clinical MR service. Factors affecting safety relate to the condition of the patient, the surrounding environment, penetration of fields through walls and the effects on staff and visitors. Bioeffects can be thermal or athermal and the science is far from being understood, although there are statements of good practice that inform the user.

Concerning MR safety (true or false)
    a. Increasing the flip angle increases the SAR.
    b. The SAR depends on the patient who is being scanned.
    c. A high SAR leads to peripheral nerve stimulation.
    d. Reducing gradient slew rates reduces peripheral nerve stimulation.
    e. Some cerebral aneurysm clips are MR safe.

Answers

a. Increasing the flip angle increases the SAR.

True: The flip angle refers to the duration of the RF pulse and is so called due to the fact that the RF can be considered to be rotating the net magnetization vector (NMV). For large flip angles the RF must be kept on for longer durations and the SAR will therefore rise.

b. The SAR depends on the patient being scanned.

True: The calculation of SAR takes into account the power of the transmitter and also the patient's mass and takes units of $W\ kg^{-1}$. For a given power being absorbed, smaller patients will therefore have an increased SAR and this is an important consideration in paediatric scanning.

c. A high SAR leads to peripheral nerve stimulation.

False: The SAR relates to RF absorption and apart from some theoretical athermal effects, the main cause of concern is heating. Nerve stimulation arises from induced currents especially in peripheral regions and occurs as a result of rapidly changing magnetic fields which is usually associated with the gradients switching.

d. Reducing gradient slew rates reduces peripheral nerve stimulation.

True: Nerve induction occurs as a result of electrical signals being inducted by rapidly changing gradient fields. If the patient or staff suspects that this may compromise safety or comfort, then the gradients' rate of change (or slew rate) can be modified.

e. Some cerebral aneurysm clips are MR safe.

True: Many metal implants are absolutely contraindicated due to magnetic forces that may cause them to move. However, some metals do not generate a magnetic force and hence are safe. It should be remembered that implants, whilst safe, may have eddy currents generated in them that distort the field and cause susceptibility artefacts or generate heat.

Q7.17 Magnetic resonance controlled area

As with x-ray imaging and many other modalities, the creation and management of a controlled area is central to establishing safe practice. The boundaries of the area must be calculated from well established principles and entry and exit from the area must be rigorously controlled. Apart from human safety, the controlled area also prevents damage to equipment which may suffer from exposure to RF or magnetic fields.

Concerning the controlled area (true or false)
a. The controlled area is the same as for x-ray imaging.
b. Pregnancy is an absolute contraindication to MR scanning.
c. A cochlear implant is a contraindication to MR scanning.
d. The controlled area can extend into the room above the magnet.
e. The inner controlled area should exclude people with pacemakers.

Answers

a. The controlled area is the same as for x-ray imaging.

False: The controlled area is designed to reduce the risk to staff, patients and visitors and must be created to reflect understanding of the risk origin. In x-ray imaging the risk arises from exposure to ionizing radiation and such risk is removed by turning off the x-ray equipment or by adequate screening. In MRI, the magnetic field remains present at all times and the field can also penetrate walls and floors/roofs leading to the need for careful surveys.

b. Pregnancy is an absolute contraindication to MR scanning.

False: Although the bioeffects of exposure to MRI are not fully understood, the technique is non-ionizing and does not introduce interactions that are not routinely encountered, although at lower intensities. Good practice demands caution, especially during the first trimester, but there is no evidence that patients have experienced harm from MRI.

c. A cochlear implant is a contraindication to MR scanning.

True: Cochlear implants use embedded electronics and metal conductors to induce sound sensations to the cochlea. The risk to the patient and to the device are significant from both magnetic force and also heating, and the device is therefore currently incompatible with MR scanning. Future developments using MR compatible materials may lead to devices which are MR safe.

d. The controlled area can extend into the room above the magnet.

True: The magnetic field extends out in all three dimensions and could well extend into the room above. A survey of the main magnetic field should be carried out on installation of the scanner and a report and diagram of the inner controlled area developed.

e. The inner controlled area should exclude people with pacemakers.

True: The inner controlled area is defined by the 0.5 mT (5 gauss) and people (staff, visitors and patients) with a pacemaker should not have access to this area. Note that the controlled area may extend outside an external wall and this area should be cordoned off.

Q7.18 Risks associated with magnetic resonance imaging

The management of safety in MR is crucial and the employer and user are responsible for ensuring the safety of all who enter the magnet environment. Image © 2013 Samuel Opoku, William Antwi, Stephanie Ruby Sarblah. Originally published in Opoku S, Antwi W and Sarblah S R 2013 Imaging and Radioanalytical Techniques in Interdisciplinary Research—Fundamentals and Cutting Edge Applications, chapter 3, under CCBY 3.0 licence. Available from http://dx.doi.org/10.5772/52699.

Concerning MR safety (true or false)
   a. There is a legal obligation to define a controlled area.
   b. Cryogens present a toxic hazard.
   c. Athermal effects present the greatest hazard to the patient.
   d. The main magnet field strength presents a major source of hazard.
   e. Active shielding fully eliminates the risk from the main magnetic field.

Answers

a. There is a legal obligation to define a controlled area.

False: The legal obligation is to ensure the establishment of safe practice in a safe area. This is conventionally achieved by the creation of a controlled area. There is a European drive to ensure a controlled area has the same status as in ionizing radiation imaging so this answer may change in the near future.

b. Cryogens present a toxic hazard.

False: The most common cryogens are liquid nitrogen and liquid helium. Both of these are non-toxic but they do displace oxygen and are considered to be a significant risk. Their mechanism of risk is asphyxia rather than toxicity.

c. Athermal effects present the greatest hazard to the patient.

False: Athermal hazards may exist as a result of RF or magnetic field exposure, but there is currently no convincing evidence that this is the case. The major risk is from the RF radiation, but a risk also arises from the magnetic field.

d. The main magnet field strength presents a major source of hazard.

True: The hazard is real and significant. There are various mechanisms for the risk, which include the ballistic effect from ferrous objects attracted to the magnet as well as the disruption of medical devices from magnetic field corruption.

e. Active shielding fully eliminates the risk from the main magnetic field.

False: An active shield utilizes a second magnetic field that is opposite in orientation to the main field. The effect of this is to partially cancel out the main field and thereby reduce its impact on the surrounding environment. However, the extent of the stray field is reduced rather than cancelled.

Q7.19 Magnetic resonance safety II

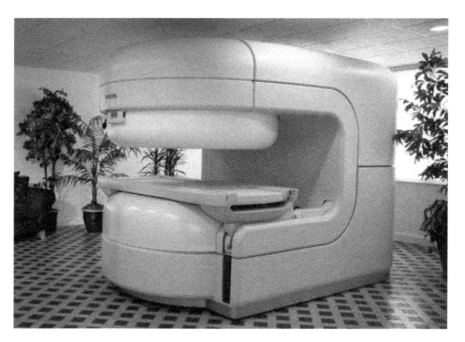

MRI has proven to be a major advance in imaging, partly as a result of its variable contrast but also because it is non-ionizing in nature which makes it safe to use. There are many field strengths, designs and applications that extend to high field magnets, MR spectroscopy and open field magnets. Open field magnets permit interventions and studies that are otherwise difficult or impossible in a closed bore magnet, but do have problems of their own.

Concerning MR safety (true or false)
 a. Open magnets present little hazard to the patient by virtue of their design.
 b. Field strengths in excess of 3 T are only available for use by special permission.
 c. Implanted ferrous materials are a significant source of hazard.
 d. The Faraday cage is designed to significantly reduce the impact of stray environmental RF.
 e. The risks to staff and patients within the MRI room are identical.

Answers
a. Open magnets present little hazard to the patient by virtue of their design.
False: Open field magnets do present a safety concern like any other MRI system and may be more difficult to risk assess as a result of their variety of uses, which includes MR guided surgery. They tend to be lower field which may reduce the main field hazard.

b. Field strengths in excess of 3 T are only available for use by special permission.
False: Fields up to 7 T are available, especially for research or small parts imaging. A case needs to be made reflecting the different risk from the higher RF. Managing bioeffects also presents problems of a different nature but these risks are accounted for during the justification stage.

c. Implanted ferrous materials are a significant source of hazard.
True: Such materials will distort the local field giving rise to susceptibility artefacts, but they can also move as a result of the force of attraction from the main field. The risk does depend on where the metal object is but the consequence can be fatal.

d. The Faraday cage is designed to significantly reduce the impact of stray environmental RF.
True: The Faraday cage is a mesh that surrounds the room and is continuous across windows and is embedded in the door structure. The mesh is sufficiently small to prevent RF from the MRI scanner affecting the surrounding environment but its major use is to prevent environmental and stray RF fields being picked up by the RF antennae and corrupting the image.

e. The risks to staff and patients within the MRI room are identical.
False: Risks to staff and patient do differ for a variety of reasons. The patient is exposed to the RF whereas the staff generally are not, and even if staff to receive RF it is usually for short durations. Staff will also have health screening and also have to declare the absence of any embedded objects.

Q7.20 Magnetic resonance imaging environment

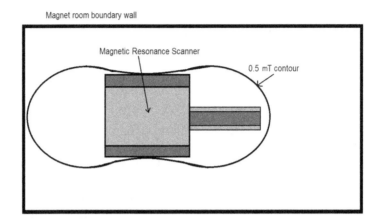

The MR environment is defined as the three-dimensional space surrounding the MR magnet that contains both the Faraday shield and the 0.5 mT contour. Anyone entering the MR environment must be screened by an MR authorised person possibly with the use of a metal detector but always using a questionnaire. Anyone seeking entry to the MR environment must be warned of the possible hazards of the magnetic field, including its impact on implanted devices and the projectile effect on ferromagnetic materials.

The MR environment (true or false)
    a. Is contained within the 0.5 mT magnetic field contour.
    b. Contains the Faraday shielded volume.
    c. Allows equipment that is MR conditional to be brought into the magnet room.
    d. Is an area where members of the public are not allowed to enter.
    e. Is accessible to carers of patients who do not require screening.

Answers

a. Is contained within the 0.5 mT magnetic field contour.

   False: The MR environment is defined as 'the three-dimensional volume of space surrounding the MR magnet that contains both the Faraday shielded volume and the 0.5 mT field contour' (by the UK Medicines and Healthcare products Regulatory Agency).

b. Contains the Faraday shielded volume.

   True: See the above definition of the MR environment.

c. Allows equipment that is MR conditional to be brought into the magnet room.

   True: Equipment that is MR conditional is defined as an item with demonstrated safety in the MR environment within defined conditions (by UK Medicines and Healthcare products Regulatory Agency).

d. Is an area where members of the public are not allowed to enter.

   True: Members of the public must be excluded from gaining access within the 0.5 mT contour.

e. Is accessible to carers of patients who do not require screening.

   False: Carers of patients may have access to the MR environment; however, they must be screened using an MR safety checklist in the same way patients are screened.

Q7.21 Magnetic resonance safety III

With regards to safety in an MR unit, an MR authorised person (supervisor) has free access to the MR environment and can supervise other staff, for example, radiographers, radiologists and clinical scientists. They will ensure that other MR authorised staff have appropriate training and awareness of their responsibilities for all other people entering the unit. During their visit to the MR centre any unauthorised staff and visitors must be under the supervision of an MR authorised person who can carry out the MR screening process. An MR operator is someone who is fully trained in the operation of the MR scanner (radiographers), however, operators may be deemed as clinical or technical (in the case of clinical scientists) who may be carrying out research.

With regards to MR safety management, an MR authorised person (true or false)
    a. Can be members of the public.
    b. Can be a patient.
    c. May be a member of staff who has not been screened for safety.
    d. May enter the MR controlled access area.
    e. May not always be allowed to enter the MR environment.

Answers

   a. Can be members of the public.

     False: All authorised personnel should be conversant with, and be able to put into practice, the general rules and emergency procedures of the MR environment.

   b. Can be a patient.

     False: See the above answer.

   c. May be a member of staff who has not been screened for safety.

     False: Authorised personnel are classified as to their level of training and will have completed a screening questionnaire.

   d. May enter the MR controlled access area.

     True: See the above answer regarding MR safety screening.

   e. May not always be allowed to enter the MR environment.

     True: There are several circumstances where an authorised person may not enter the MR environment, for example, pregnancy.

Q7.22 Magnetic resonance safety IV

Any ferromagnetic
object is at risk

Coins, gas cylinders, keys, paper clips,
hospital beds, credit cards, chairs,
infusion pumps, scissors.

Iron, cobalt and nickel based objects

There are four main types of hazard in an MR environment. These hazards arise from the static magnetic field, the time varying magnetic fields (gradients), the RF delivery system and acoustic noise. The static magnetic field can create a projectile effect on any ferromagnetic object (that is materials containing iron, cobalt or nickel). The projectile effect is so strong that it easily attracts objects like gas cylinders or floor burnishers. Gradient magnetic fields can cause peripheral neural stimulation. Radiofrequency electromagnetic fields can cause heating and MR systems are calibrated to calculate the specific absorption rate for a pulse sequence. Acoustic noise within the MR environment is caused by the switching gradient magnetic fields and hearing protection can be provided.

Concerning safety within an MR scanner (true or false)
a. The most common cause of adverse incidents in MR is claustrophobia.
b. Radiofrequency fields can induce electric currents in conducting wires and cause them to heat up.
c. Anatomy, for example limbs, that form a conductive loop may be at risk of burning in an MR scanner.
d. A rise of 3 °C in body temperature is acceptable in a normal person.
e. Time varying magnetic fields pose no risks in MR scanning.

Answers

a. The most common cause of adverse incidents in MR is claustrophobia.

False: Claustrophobia does occur in MRI scanning, however, with correct patient screening it can be reduced dramatically. The most common adverse incident is patients or staff possessing some form of metal in the magnet room.

b. Radiofrequency fields can induce electric currents in conducting wires and cause them to heat up.

True: Wires associated with patient monitoring equipment can be a cause for concern due to RF induction heating with the risk of stress induced current burns and contact burns.

c. Anatomy, for example limbs, that form a conductive loop may be at risk of burning in an MR scanner.

True: Conductive loops, especially in the limbs should be avoided using foam pads placed where there are areas of touching skin.

d. A rise of 3 °C in body temperature is acceptable in a normal person.

False: A temperature rise of 1 °C is generally acceptable in a normal healthy person.

e. Time varying magnetic fields pose no risks in MR scanning.

False: Time varying magnetic fields (magnetic field gradients) may cause biological effects, peripheral nerve stimulation, muscle stimulation and pose a risk due to acoustic noise.

Q7.23 Gradient echo imaging

There are two families of pulse sequences in MR imaging. These are the spin echo sequences which use a 180° RF pulse to create the MR signal (echo) and gradient echo pulse sequences which use gradient magnetic fields to create the MR signal. Gradient magnetic fields can be applied more rapidly than an RF pulse to create the MR signal and therefore the gradient sequences are able to employ shorter echo times (TE). As a result of this, gradient echo sequences can be programmed to work more rapidly. A disadvantage (or advantage) of gradient echo sequences is that they produce images of T2* weighting rather than pure T2.

Gradient echo imaging in MRI (true or false)
a. Produces images of T1 or T2* weighting.
b. Uses very short repetition times, TR = 20 ms.
c. Rephasing of protons is achieved using a 180° RF pulse.
d. The MR signal is generated using two magnetic field gradients.
e. In general, uses a flip angle greater than 90°.

Answers

a. Produces images of T1 or T2* weighting.

True: The gradient echo pulse sequence can produce T1 and T2* weighted images depending on choice of TR, TE and flip angle. It cannot produce pure T2 weighted images due to the presence of magnetic field inhomogeneities.

b. Uses very short repetition times, typically, TR = 20 ms.

True: Very short TR times are used with even shorter TE times.

c. Rephasing of protons is achieved using a 180° RF pulse.

False: Rephasing of protons is achieved by the application of a dephasing followed by a rephasing magnetic field gradient. A spin echo pulse sequence uses a 180° RF pulse.

d. The MR signal is generated using two magnetic field gradients.

True: The gradient echo (MR signal) is created by the application of a dephasing gradient, followed by a rephasing gradient.

e. In general, uses a flip angle greater than 90°.

False: In general, uses flip angles less than 90°, this enables shorter TR and TE times to be used.

Q7.24 Magnetic resonance imaging spatial encoding

The MR signal is received in the RF coils that are placed close to the patient's anatomy. The body is repeatedly energised and an MR signal recorded multiple times. At each excitation differing spatial encoding is applied. Spatial encoding is carried out using gradient magnetic fields in each of the x-, y- and z-directions. A gradient applied perpendicular to the plane of acquisition is termed the slice select gradient. Gradient magnetic fields within the plane are termed the frequency and phase encoding gradients.

In magnetic resonance imaging spatial encoding (true or false)
a. Axial/transverse slices are selected by a z-gradient.
b. Pixels within the image are encoded by two co-ordinates (phase and frequency).
c. Generates thinner slices with a weaker gradient.
d. Creates varying Larmor frequencies along a magnetic field gradient.
e. Uses a narrow band of RF to excite a thin slice of tissue.

Answers

a. Axial/transverse slices are selected by a z-gradient.

   True: The z-gradient (and axis within an MR scanner) is traditionally applied along the long axis of the body, from head to foot, and this selects transverse slices.

b. Pixels within the image are encoded by two co-ordinates (phase and frequency).

   True: The x- and y-axes of the MR image are encoded using frequency and phase encoding gradients in these directions, however, these may be reversed.

c. Generates thinner slices with a weaker gradient.

   False: A stronger magnetic field gradient is required to select a thinner slice.

d. Creates varying Larmor frequencies along a magnetic field gradient.

   True: The Larmor frequency of the precessing protons increases with increasing magnetic field and reduces with lower magnetic field.

e. Uses a narrow band of RF to excite a thin slice of tissue.

   True: A narrow band RF pulse can be used to generate a thin slice, whilst a broader band RF pulse will select a thicker slice.

Q7.25 Magnetic resonance signal

During MR imaging slices of the body are energised using a 90° RF pulse. This is a short burst of RF radiation (1–5 ms) which is absorbed by hydrogen protons within water and fat tissue. After the RF pulse is switched off, the energy that was absorbed begins to be released. The energy is released in several ways and takes varying times (relaxation times), depending on the tissue type, local magnetic and molecular environment. MR imaging exploits the difference in these relaxation times between different tissues and disease within the body.

Concerning the magnetic resonance signal (true or false)
a. T1 relaxation times are generally shorter than T2 relaxation times.
b. Spin–lattice relaxation (T1) is due to proton interaction with their molecular environment.
c. Spin–spin relaxation (T2) results in the loss of phase coherence.
d. Tissues which are more solid (bone, calculi, teeth) have very long T2.
e. Variation in T1 and T2 is greater than proton density throughout the body.

Answers

   a. T1 relaxation times are generally shorter than T2 relaxation times.

      False: The opposite is true, T2 relaxation times are generally much shorter than T1.

   b. Spin–lattice relaxation (T1) is due to proton interaction with their molecular environment.

      True: Spin-lattice relaxation causes the proton magnetic moments to return to their equilibrium position precessing around the main magnetic field. Energy is transferred from the excited protons (energised by a 90° RF pulse) to their surrounding environment, referred to as a lattice.

   c. Spin–spin relaxation (T2) results in the loss of phase coherence.

      True: After the absorption of energy through the 90° RF pulse, protons interact with local magnetic fields inhomogeneities (variations generated by neighbouring protons). This causes the protons to precess at differing frequencies which in turn causes them to get out of alignment with each other. This increasing lack of alignment is called incoherence.

   d. Tissues which are more solid (bone, calculi, teeth) have very long T2.

      False: Tissues that are more solid have shorter T2 times and therefore the MR signal decays very rapidly within them, to the extent that it is difficult to collect any MR signal.

   e. Variation in T1 and T2 is greater than proton density throughout the body.

      True: Variation of proton density within the body is approximately 10% within the body, whereas T1 and T2 vary by much greater amounts. Therefore, we get increased image contrast when the MR signal is based on the differences in T1 or T2 times compared to proton density.

IOP Publishing

Scientific Basis of the Royal College of Radiologists Fellowship (2nd Edition)

Illustrated questions and answers

Malcolm Sperrin and John Winder

Chapter 8

Nuclear medicine

Nuclear medicine or RNI (Radionuclide Imaging) is a specialist but highly valuable technique in that it images tissue function rather than anatomy to define presentation of image contrast. It generally requires the administration of unsealed radioactive sources which makes the management of radiation protection fairly complex. The dose to the patient also differs from that given to patients during CT for instance in that the radiation provides a systemic exposure that is present for some time after the imaging procedure has finished. There are many manifestations of RNI including hybrid imaging where the final image is a combination of anatomical and functional imaging that generates a fused image that is very useful for the clinical staging of some diseases.

doi:10.1088/978-0-7503-2148-8ch8

Q8.1 Gamma camera design

The gamma camera is sometimes know as the Anger camera. This latter term arises as a result of the type of logic used to create the final image but the term gamma camera is now almost uniquely used. The whole premise of the camera is that it converts gamma rays into an image and because the rays have no charge and cannot be easily bent like light, there needs to be a more ingenious method of spatial localization. Furthermore, the conversion of the gammas to elements of the image is also complex and presents complexities of its own.

Concerning the gamma camera (true or false)
   a. Without the collimator, no image can be created.
   b. Sodium iodide (NaI) crystals are used as scintillators because they are most efficient at 140 keV.
   c. The count rate is limited primarily by the decoding circuitry.
   d. The gamma camera can be used to detect two gamma energies concurrently.
   e. Only gammas entering through the collimator will contribute to the final image.

Answers

a. Without the collimator, no image can be created.

False: The conversion of gammas to light and then to a component of the image will still occur but the resolution will be poor. The collimator enables the direction of the incoming gamma to be determined and hence without it there will be a large acceptance angle making the origin of the gamma uncertain. The resolution that arises without the collimator in place is due to the finite size of the PM tubes.

b. NaI crystals are used as scintillators because they are most efficient at 140 keV.

True: NaI absorbs gammas and the energy is converted into visible light. This process depends upon the absorbance of the NaI and also its arrangement of energy levels which makes it sensitive to certain wavelengths or energies. Although NaI can be used at other energies, its efficiency is reduced. Because Technetium (Tc) is so widely used and has a photo peak at 140 keV, NaI, which absorbs strongly at this energy, is also widely used.

c. The count rate is limited primarily by the decoding circuitry.

False: The electronic circuitry can be a limiting factor but the crystal has a saturation effect where the arrival of two gammas very closely together are not identified as separate events. This is most easily seen when the peaks associated with the gamma rays fully overlap, they will only register as a single event. The two arrivals must have sufficient separation and hence this will relate to the count rate.

d. The gamma camera can be used to detect two gamma energies concurrently.

True: The detector and associated electronics can discriminate between energies provided that there is sufficient energy difference between the gammas. The choice of energy window makes this possible and is also used to discriminate between incident gammas and scatter.

e. Only gammas entering through the collimator will contribute to the final image.

True: Ambient gammas can be a problem in some investigations and the gamma camera is shielded to significantly reduce unwanted stray gammas contributing to noise in the final image.

Q8.2 The ideal isotope

Table 8.1. Radioactive isotopes used for metastatic bone pain management.

Isotope	Emission	Mean half-life (days)	Mean β energy (keV)	Soft tissue penetration (mm)
Phosphorus (^{23}P)	β	14.4	695	8
Strontium (^{89}Sr)	β	50.5	583	2.4
Samarium (^{153}Sm)	β and γ	18.6	233	3.1
Renium (^{186}Re)	β and γ	3.8	349	1.1
Tin (^{117}Sn)	β and γ	13.6	135	0.3

Radioactive isotopes have characteristics that make them desirable for imaging but can also present limitations to the imaging process whether as a result of radiation dose, attenuation and availability. The choice of isotope is therefore, limited although there is active research to identify uses where less common isotopes can be bound to pharmaceuticals for new techniques. An ideal radionuclide for imaging purposes should have a short physical half-life (a few hours) so that it is active within the body during the imaging time; it should decay by emission of gamma rays only (alpha or beta particles contribute to patient dose but not the image); it should decay to a stable nuclide daughter; the gamma rays should be mono-energetic and in the range 50–300 keV.

Concerning the ideal isotope (true or false)
   a. The ideal isotope for imaging has no particulate emission.
   b. Long half-life isotopes are favoured because they permit rescans without the need for further injection of radioactivity.
   c. The isotope is chosen for its ability to locate at an organ of choice.
   d. Tc is often used because it is relatively easily converted to light by the scintillator.
   e. Toxic isotopes can be used provided they are approved through the IRMER process.

Answers

a. The ideal isotope for imaging has no particulate emission.

True: The usual particle to accompany gamma emission is the beta particle. This contributes to the dose to the patient and has no part to play in the imaging. Particle emission is therefore to be avoided.

b. Long half-life isotopes are favoured because they permit rescans without the need for further injection of radioactivity.

True: However a lot involved in this question. If an isotope has a very short half-life a repeat scan would necessitate a further administration of the isotope and thus increase the dose. If the activity is too long then the patient remains radioactive for a long duration, thus irradiating themselves and others again with negative effects. The general guidance is that the ideal isotope should have a half-life comparable to the duration of the study and hence Tc, with its half-life of 6 hours is a good choice.

c. The isotope is chosen for its ability to locate at an organ of choice.

False: It is the carrier drug that will cause the localization. The same isotope can be used for a variety of different studies or different isotopes for the same study.

d. Tc is often used because it is relatively easily converted to light by the scintillator.

True: Whilst true, there are other reasons why Tc is suitable, such as its half-life, convenient chemistry, ease of manufacture, etc.

e. Toxic isotopes can be used provided they are approved through the IRMER process.

False: IRMER relates to radiation control and management and is not part of the process to establish chemical safety.

Q8.3 Quality assurance tests

Any imaging system requires assessment to ensure that it is fit for purpose as well as making sure that patient safety is not compromised. Image uniformity, spatial resolution and energy resolution are important factors to check on a regular basis. A flood field (generated by a single radiation source far away from the gamma camera face) will provide a near uniform exposure across the gamma camera detector to test photomultiplier response. Background radiation checks will indicate any contamination or the presence of unshielded sources near the camera. Blurring within the gamma camera is caused by a number of factors including the statistical nature of radiation detection, radiation scatter within the patient and light scatter within the sodium iodide crystal. Improved energy resolution, the ability to separate out different gamma ray energies, allows improved removal of scatter and therefore improved spatial resolution.

Concerning QA tests
    a. QA is not an urgent requirement in radionuclide imaging because the resolution is so poor.
    b. Daily QA commonly includes the uniformity assessment.
    c. The PM tubes only need to be checked upon commissioning because, being electronic, they are very stable long term.
    d. Count rate and sensitivity are checked on a regular basis.
    e. The energy acceptance window has an effect on the noise within the image.

Answers

    a. QA is not an urgent requirement in radionuclide imaging because the resolution is so poor.

        False: QA may assess resolution but it also assesses contrast and consistency. It is important to know all of these factors and consistency checks are often overlooked by the candidate. Consistency will ensure that a view taken on one occasion should be the same some time later if the patient's condition does not change.

    b. Daily QA commonly includes the uniformity assessment.

        True: Uniformity ensures that all parts of the gamma camera head are equally sensitive. Electronic drift or degrading components can have an effect on uniformity and these can change on a scale of hours to and hence a daily check with a flood phantom is often called for.

    c. The PM tubes only need to be checked upon commissioning because, being electronic, they are very stable long term.

        False: PM tubes are electronic amplifiers and can drift significantly with time and ageing. If their gain does change then the image can develop dark or light regions which interfere with the overall appearance of the image.

    d. Count rate and sensitivity are checked on a regular basis.

        True: The count rate is a function of administered activity, collimation and sensitivity and all are relevant to the imaging process and can be used to inform the dose to the patient. The sensitivity can be measured by use of a known activity. Both are tested as part of an on-going QA programme.

    e. The energy acceptance window has an effect on the noise within the image.

        True: The energy peak as detected and measured by the gamma camera will be much broader than that of the undetected gamma. This arises due to scatter and hence the influence of scatter on the final image can be reduced by being selective of the energy range accepted for imaging.

Q8.4 Dynamic studies

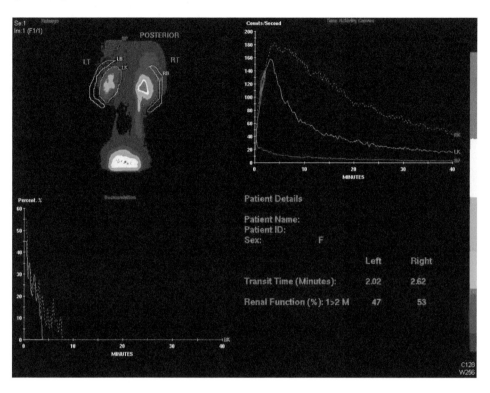

Dynamic nuclear medicine imaging may use radioisotopes to assess tissue function and the function associated with metastases or lung and will not vary significantly over short time periods, making time-resolved imaging possible. For studies investigating the function of the kidney the change in radioactivity over time is monitored as the isotope reaches the kidney and subsequently is excreted. The uptake into the kidney, the transit through the kidney and the elimination of the tracer from the kidney provide evidence as to its function. This requires a time resolved acquisition in that images are acquired over a period of 20–30 minutes. Such dynamic scans acquire counts for a set time period from a given region.

Concerning dynamic studies (true or false)
a. Dynamic studies tend to be qualitative rather than quantitative.
b. The background needs to be taken into account when assessing renal function using isotopes.
c. Radioactive urine shows up as a hot spot on the renogram.
d. Count rates of a few thousand per second are sufficient for dynamic renograms.
e. Temporal resolutions of minutes are common.

Answers

a. Dynamic studies tend to be qualitative rather than quantitative.

False: Quantification is possible even if not always fully utilized. Count rate rather than just sensitivity is important which makes the assessment of function possible as in the case of dynamic studies. Quantification can also be used to assess dose and its distribution, assuming the activity, uptake, etc, are known.

b. The background needs to be taken into account when assessing renal function using isotopes.

True: When the renal function is assessed, the activity of the tissue over and underlying the kidney needs to be taken into account. This is usually achieved by subtracting an area of background activity adjacent to but separate from the kidney.

c. Radioactive urine shows up as a hot spot on the renogram.

True: Whilst the change in activity within the visible bounds of the kidney are used to asses renal function, the pooling of radioactive urine in the bladder does give rise to a significant hot spot. The bladder can be sufficiently active to dominate the available grey scale and hence is sometimes shielded to permit the more accurate windowing of the grey scale from the kidneys.

d. Count rates of a few thousand per second are sufficient for dynamic renograms.

True: Count rate variations as the isotope passes through the kidney range from a few tens of thousands to a few hundred depending upon the stage of excretion or the duration of the acquisition.

e. Temporal resolutions of minutes are common.

False: The temporal resolution is usually measured in seconds which permits the accurate display of changes over periods of minutes. The temporal resolution can be imagined to be the duration of the discrete activity measurement. This is divided up into short periods called bins.

Q8.5 Nuclear medicine risks

1980

2006

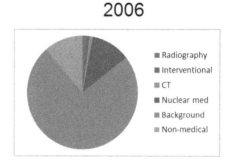

Radiation dose to the patient is inevitable in nuclear medicine as the radionuclide is taken up by a specific organ which in turn acts as a radiation source. Other nearby tissues will become irradiated by the source organ. The dose to an organ will depend on the effective half-life of the activity within the organ, the amount of the activity actually taken up by the organ, the original activity administered and the energies of the gamma radiation and other radiation emitted during decay. Radiation will also be taken away from the organ by natural processes and eventually excreted.

Concerning nuclear medicine safety (true or false)
  a. Nuclear medicine dose has increased as a result of more complex treatments.
  b. The primary risk from nuclear medicine is that associated with radiation exposure.
  c. Doses of in excess of 10 mSv are common for bone scans.
  d. Nuclear medicine imaging is absolutely contraindicated during pregnancy.
  e. One foetal dose is of major concern during nuclear medicine exams even if imaging the brain of the mother.

Answers

a. Nuclear medicine dose has increased as a result of more complex treatments.

False: The use of nuclear medicine provides insight into the location of elevated metabolism and whilst complex treatments may use the data so obtained, its use is not significantly increasing beyond that associated with a growing population. Other imaging options are increasing where, for instance, new contrast options are introduced.

b. The primary risk from nuclear medicine is that associated with radiation exposure.

True: The radiation exposure in nuclear medicine is significant and must be justified as for any radiation based investigation. There are, however, other risks such as that from poor tolerance of the pharmaceuticals but these are rare. It is also important to understand that the risk is systemic rather than localized since the isotopes are injected and remain circulating until they are excreted or decay.

c. Doses of in excess of 10 mSv are common for bone scans.

False: Typical doses vary between patients and centres, but 1–4 mSv is a reasonably representative value.

d. Nuclear medicine imaging is absolutely contraindicated during pregnancy.

False: The referring clinician needs to exercise caution over the concerns for non-pregnant patients, but actions can be taken to reduce dose where a nuclear medicine investigation is called for. Ventilation only scans for instance instead of ventilation quotient scans or the use of reduced activity.

e. Foetal dose is of major concern during nuclear medicine exams even if imaging the brain of the mother.

True: Dose is always a concern whether to staff or patient. Furthermore, since nuclear medicine usually requires an isotope to be injected, the radiation becomes systemic, leading to a does to the foetus irrespective of the original site of investigation.

Q8.6 Positron emission tomography I

Positron emission tomography (PET) permits the creation of a tomographic image based on tissue function. The most common positron emitter used in medicine is ^{18}F which emits a positive beta particle. This positron travels a short distance through the body when emitted (~2 mm) before being annihilated by an electron (−ve). The annihilation results in the production of two 511 keV gamma rays which are used to help form the image. The gamma rays which are essential to the image formation arise from annihilation processes which are preferentially located in tissue of elevated fluorine uptake. Isotopes which eject positrons are generated in a cyclotron and are usually of short half-life making their transport and utilization more challenging that for conventional isotopes. Glucose analogues such as fluorodeoxyglucose (FDG) are routinely used.

Concerning PET imaging (true or false)
  a. PET utilizes the coincident arrival of two electrons.
  b. Resolution decreases if isotopes generating high energy positrons are used.
  c. Gammas emitted from an annihilation event are always ejected exactly 180° apart.
  d. PET resolution is comparable to that of the gamma camera.
  e. Collimation is not essential for PET scans.

Answers
 a. PET utilizes the coincident arrival of two electrons.
   False: It is the arrival of two gammas that is recorded in coincidence. The gammas are ejected from an annihilation reaction between a positron and an electron. The positron is from the decay of the isotope and the electron found naturally in the tissue. In order to conserve momentum, the gammas are almost opposite in direction.
 b. Resolution decreases if isotopes generating high energy positrons are used.
   True: The most intuitive answer here is that the positron will travel further if it has more energy and hence greater velocity. Since the original direction of travel of the positron is random, this equates to a volume of uncertainty thus affecting resolution since the origin of the annihilation becomes uncertain.
 c. Gammas emitted from an annihilation event are always ejected exactly 180° apart.
   False: They can vary by very small angles and this will affect the uncertainty in origin of the annihilation event. The variation from perfect opposition arises due to the momentum of the positron which must be conserved and appears as inhomogeneity in the gamma direction.
 d. PET resolution is comparable to that of the gamma camera.
   True: It is comparable to the gamma camera, being around $4\,\mathrm{lp\ cm^{-1}}$.
 e. Collimation is not essential for PET scans.
   True: The reason for this is that the only events that will contribute to the final image are those detected in opposition and coincidence, meaning that no collimation is needed between the detectors.

Q8.7 Single photon emission computed tomography I

Single photon emission CT (SPECT) is another isotope based imaging technique used in nuclear medicine which relies upon the use of two or more gamma cameras. The technique permits the creation of tomographic images from planar detectors and in this sense it is comparable to how CT works. The gantry containing the gamma camera heads rotates around the patient collecting emission profiles of gamma rays, perhaps up to 30 seconds per view and requires about 30 minutes to complete data acquisition. Image reconstruction is by filtered back projection. The range of applications is increasing but it is most familiar in use for cardiac and neurological studies.

Concerning SPECT (true or false)
- a. SPECT utilizes at least three gamma cameras.
- b. SPECT is a useful tool to image cardiac muscle function.
- c. SPECT does not require collimation to form an image.
- d. NAI scintillators are commonly used in the detection process.
- e. SPECT systems have a dynamic facility to ensure the detectors are as close to the patient as possible.

Answers

a. SPECT utilizes at least three gamma cameras.

False: SPECT only requires two cameras to be able to generate the image. Three cameras can be used which increases the count statistics and can reduce the duration of the imaging process. The orientation of the cameras, whether in opposition or at 90°, etc, is one of design rather than based on physical principles.

b. SPECT is a useful tool to image cardiac muscle function.

True: This is one of the major applications. SPECT enables tomographic images to be generated from a variety of directions permitting the identification of defects.

c. SPECT does not require collimation to form an image.

False: Whilst data can be collected without the collimator in place, the resulting image would be of such poor quality as to be largely without clinical value. The gamma camera requires a collimator for precisely the same reasons as the conventional gamma camera.

d. NAI scintillators are commonly used in the detection process.

True: This is the same as for a planar gamma camera.

e. SPECT systems have a dynamic facility to ensure the detectors are as close to the patient as possible.

True: The image quality can be degraded by the presence of a large gap between the detector and the patient whereby the gammas continue to diverge and decrease resolution and contrast. The individual gamma heads are automatically controlled so as to reduce the gap, consistent with the safety and comfort of the patient.

Q8.8 Combined positron emission tomography/computed tomography

PET/CT is one of the original hybrid imaging techniques where functional and anatomical information can be displayed together. Hybrid imaging, combining data from two or more imaging systems, does introduce some reconstruction problems such as the vital need for correct registration between images and this is achieved in a number of different ways. Hybrid imaging is a major advance in that it permits regions of tissue to be associated with elevated metabolism and as such is a useful staging tool.

In PET/CT (true or false)
    a. In a PET/CT system, the attenuation properties of the tissue can be determined to improve the contrast of the PET image.
    b. Radiation administered during the CT phase is also used for the PET phase.
    c. Large uncertainties arise as a result of the image overlay process.
    d. The radiation from the PET isotope contributes to noise in the CT image.
    e. Artefacts arise from beam hardening.

Answers

a. In a PET/CT system, the attenuation properties of the tissue can be determined to improve the contrast of the PET image.

True: The gammas originating as part of the PET imaging process will be
attenuated by the tissue through which they pass. The attenuation can be
approximated by the CT process which uses the attenuation as a basis for
the final CT image. The correction is not exact since the attenuation and
correction are derived from different photon energies.

b. Radiation administered during the CT phase is also used for the PET phase.

False: The radiation associated with the CT element is different in energy,
type and administration from that used in the PET component. The
reason for them being hybridized is one of efficiency of process.

c. Large uncertainties arise as a result of the image overlay process.

False: Great care is taken to ensure that the images are properly
co-registered. The implications of associating a functional hotspot with
the wrong anatomy is clinically extremely significant.

d. The radiation from the PET isotope contributes to noise in the CT image.

True: However, the noise from the PET process will be very small in
comparison to noise arising from CT scatter during the x-ray acquisition.
Procedures may lead to CT being conducted first with the PET injection
and imaging occurring as a second stage.

e. Artefacts arise from beam hardening.

True: Beam hardening is a well known artefact arising from the preferential absorption of low energy x-rays which results in greater penetration for the remaining higher energy x-rays. This is a part of the CT
imaging process and care is taken to minimize beam hardening artefacts.

Q8.9 Collimators

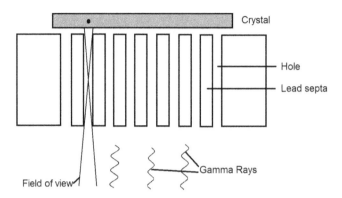

The collimator is a crucial part of the gamma camera. Its use is necessary since gamma rays cannot be focused in a manner similar to that of light or charged particles. The basic premise is that non-normal incidence gammas are likely to be associated with scatter and it is desirable to remove them. This acceptance angle is not precisely 90° since the distance to the patient is finite and hence will have an associated divergence angle. The collimator hole width, collimator thickness and holes per unit area are all important factors in determining the overall characteristics.

Concerning collimators used for nuclear medicine (true or false)
    a. High energy gammas give rise to poorer resolution for a given collimator.
    b. Resolution varies with distance from the collimator.
    c. The area occupied by the septa exceeds the area of the apertures for a general purpose collimator.
    d. High energy collimators are used for isotopes that produce gammas greater than 200 keV.
    e. Collimators only marginally affect the overall count rate.

Answers

a. High energy gammas give rise to poorer resolution for a given collimator.

   True: Higher energy gammas will be able to penetrate through a greater thicknesses of lead. The scattered radiation will therefore form a greater part of the image leading to a reduction in resolution.

b. Resolution varies with distance from the collimator.

   False: The resolution will primarily be governed by the gamma energy and collimator used. As the patient's distance to the camera increases, the acceptance angle of the collimator will not change but the radiation will appear to come form a source that behaves more like a point. This is offset by the separation and the inverse square law which combine to affect the contrast rather than resolution.

c. The area occupied by the septa exceeds the area of the apertures for a general purpose collimator.

   False: Apertures of around 1 mm and septa of around 0.2 mm are representative.

d. High energy collimators are used for isotopes that produce gammas greater than 200 keV.

   False: High energy collimators are usually associated with gamma energies above 350 keV. Tc emits gammas with an energy of 140 keV which are low energy when considering which collimator to select.

e. Collimators only marginally affect the overall count rate.

   False: Collimators will very significantly affect the count rate. The easiest way to visualize this is to consider the purpose of the collimator itself. It is designed to reduce the transmission of scattered gammas which will form a large percentage of the overall incident gammas. Removal of the collimator entirely makes this fact very evident.

Q8.10 Resolution

Spatial resolution in nuclear medicine is a significant limiting factor in its imaging performance. The resolution is limited by factors such as the collimator characteristics, gamma energy, scatter and the sodium iodide (NaI) crystal and the influence of all of these needs to be recognized and understood, especially if there is a suspicion of a system fault such as the wrong collimator or degraded PM tubes.

Concerning resolution in nuclear medicine (true or false)
    a. Resolutions of the order of 1 lp mm^{-1} are possible with gamma camera imaging.
    b. Resolution is greater for low object to collimator distances.
    c. PET and SPECT have similar resolutions.
    d. The energy acceptance window can be reduced to increase resolution.
    e. Resolutions with the collimator removed are sufficiently poor to make imaging impractical.

Answers

a. Resolutions of the order of 1 lp mm^{-1} are possible with gamma camera imaging.

   False: This is a good example of checking the units. The indicative resolution is around 1 lp cm^{-1}, i.e. a factor of 10 worse. In comparison to the CT resolution of 2 lp mm^{-1}, nuclear medicine is usually referred to as a poor resolution technique.

b. Resolution is greater for low object to collimator distances.

   False: The resolution will not be significantly affected by patient detector separation. As the patient gets closer, the divergence of the gammas will effectively increase, leading to more gammas being attenuated by the collimator. The acceptance angle of the collimator holes will, however, stay the same.

c. PET and SPECT have similar resolutions.

   True: They are similar but not same being around 1 lp cm^{-1} and 2 lp cm^{-1}, respectively.

d. The energy acceptance window can be reduced to increase resolution.

   False: This will change contrast rather than resolution since it will modify the gammas that have penetrated through the collimator already. Decreasing the energy window will reduce the counts that contribute to the image from scatter.

e. Resolutions with the collimator removed are sufficiently poor to make imaging impractical.

   True: Some types of imaging are possible but these relate largely to total counts rather than seeking the best resolution. The resolution possible without the collimator in place is a factor of ten or so worse than that with it present.

Q8.11 Bone scans

Bone scans form a significant proportion of the activity of a nuclear medicine department. The process requires an injected radiopharmaceutical that will preferentially locate on regions of elevated function which includes tumour sites, but also those areas associated with trauma and degenerative change. The site of injection can often appear to be hot, as can the filling bladder.

Concerning bone scanning (true or false)
   a. Imaging protocols have a critical effect on the efficacy of the bone scan.
   b. Fractures can mimic the uptake from the raised metabolic activity of tumours.
   c. Methylene diphosphonate (MDP) and hydroxymethylene diphosphonate (HDP) differ primarily in their carrier pharmaceutical.
   d. Typical doses are around 500 MBq.
   e. Hotspots always indicate elevated metabolic activity.

Answers

a. Imaging protocols have a critical effect on the efficacy of the bone scan.

   True: Bones scans conducted too early or too late may give rise to reduced contrast at sites where uptake is subtle. Manufacturers will state for their recommended pharmaceuticals the delay between injection and imaging which reflects the metabolic uptake at relevant sites.

b. Fractures can mimic the uptake from the raised metabolic activity of tumours.

   True: Fractures will have associated with them increased blood supply and this will be easily visualized during a bone scan. This can include stress fractures or degenerative changes and is common in the hips and lower spine.

c. MDP and HDP differ primarily in their carrier pharmaceutical.

   True: These two pharmaceuticals are competitors and differ in the pharmaceutical that is used to bring the Tc to the target organ. They also differ in the delay between administration and imaging, but the primary difference is the drug itself.

d. Typical activities are around 500 MBq.

   True: However, this is just indicative since the actual activity will vary enormously between patients, study type, etc. The ARSAC certificate awarded to a clinician will dictate the limit that it is permissible to give.

e. Hotspots always indicate elevated metabolic activity.

   False: Hotspots can also be associated with point of injection, bladder filling, surface sills, etc.

Q8.12 Photomultiplier tubes

The photomultiplier tubes used in nuclear medicine gamma cameras act as amplifiers for the light signal that has been generated in the photocathode. An incident light photon from the NaI crystal is converted into electrons in the photocathode. These photoelectrons are created at a rate of typically one electron per 10 light photons. To amplify the signal the photoelectrons are accelerated through a series of voltage stages called dynodes—the amplification is also called the 'gain'. As the electrons are accelerated they strike the dynodes and create extra electrons, in effect, creating an avalanche effect, this amplifying the signal. Photomultiplier tubes are a crucial part in the chain of detection and image formation. They tend to be large and bulky and can be prone to variations in performance that makes their routine testing important.

Concerning PM tubes used in nuclear medicine (true or false)
  a. PM tube gain can be as high as 10^5.
  b. PM tubes can suffer from drift leading to image artefacts.
  c. PM tubes are usually the most fragile component in the gamma camera.
  d. PET imaging utilizes an annular array of PM tubes.
  e. Care must be taken to ensure intimate contact between the PM tube and the scintillation crystal.

Answers

a. PM tube gain can be as high as 10^5.

True: The PM tube is a multistage process where electrons are attracted by high voltages between stages at which each electron is multiplied up. The multiplication factor depends on how many stages there are and also the excitation voltages, but 10^5 is typical.

b. PM tubes can suffer from drift leading to image artefacts.

True: Being electronic, their performance can drift from day to day and also over time. Checks on their gain and stability are important since faults can be shown on the final image as areas of unexpected brightness.

c. PM tubes are usually the most fragile component in the gamma camera.

False: The tubes are certainly fragile but other components also require great care in their handling. The NaI crystal is both fragile and sensitive to moisture which makes it the most likely item to need attention if due care is not given to looking after the gamma camera.

d. PET imaging utilizes an annular array of PM tubes.

False: The array is annular but the detectors are usually solid state.

e. Care must be taken to ensure intimate contact between the PM tube and the scintillation crystal.

True: The PM tube acts to amplify low intensity flashes from the NaI crystal and good optical coupling is essential to maximize the available signal.

Q8.13 Single photon emission computed tomography II

Conventional planar gamma camera imaging produces a two-dimensional projection of radioactivity that is distributed throughout the body. Radioactive organs and tissues are superimposed on each other within the projected image and therefore, depth information and image contrast may be lost. In SPECT imaging, a gamma camera head using a parallel hole collimator rotates around the patient collecting image data. There is significant absorption of gamma rays from deep within the body compared to those emitted close to the surface. A correction algorithm is applied for depth gamma attenuation at various depths within the body.

In single photon emission computed tomography (true or false)
    a. A single gamma camera may be used to acquire image data.
    b. There is an increase in spatial resolution over planar nuclide imaging.
    c. There is a reduction in noise compared to planar nuclide imaging.
    d. Collimation is required as in planar imaging.
    e. Coincidence detection requires the capture of two photons.

Answers

a. A single gamma camera may be used to acquire image data.

True: A single gamma camera head can collect data through a 180° rotation and produce an image.

b. There is an increase in spatial resolution over planar nuclide imaging.

False: Spatial resolution in SPECT is not as great as planar nuclide imaging, however, this is offset by an increase in image contrast resolution.

c. There is a reduction in noise compared to planar nuclide imaging.

False: There is an increase in noise in SPECT images due to the acquisition of a lower number of photons.

d. Collimation is required as in planar imaging.

True: Collimation is required in any gamma camera head to reject scattered photons and therefore improve spatial resolution.

e. Coincidence detection requires the capture of two photons.

False: Coincident detection occurs in positron emission tomography and not SPECT.

Q8.14 Positron emission tomography II

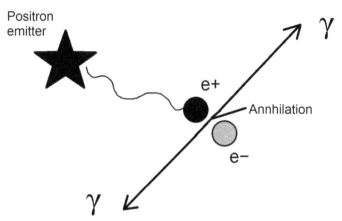

where γ is a gamma ray, e⁻ is an electron and e⁺ is a positron

The radioactive process of positron decay was discovered in 1933 and within a few years was being used in animal tracer studies. Positron emitting radionuclides require a surplus of positive charge within the nucleus and are created within a cyclotron. A cyclotron consists of two semi-circular copper electrodes contained within a vacuum and a strong magnetic field. Positively charged ions are accelerated away from the electrodes towards a target material. The radionuclides produced are generally short-lived and are therefore transferred directly to a pharmaceutical synthesis system to produce the radioactive tracer.

Regarding positron emission tomography (PET) imaging (true or false)

    a. ^{18}F emits an electron which travels 2 cm through tissue.
    b. A positron is an electron with a positive electrical charge.
    c. The process of annihilation (positron/electron combination) produces two energetic photons.
    d. 511 keV photons are emitted perpendicular to each other.
    e. Emitted photons are detected by bismuth germanate (BGO) detector.

Answers

a. ^{18}F emits an electron which travels 2 cm through tissue.

False: ^{18}F emits a positron which travels 1–2 mm within the body before annihilation.

b. A positron is an electron with a positive electrical charge.

True: Yes, a positron has the same mass but opposite charge to an electron.

c. The process of annihilation (positron/electron combination) produces two energetic photons.

True: Yes, two energetic photons are emitted in opposite directions after the annihilation process.

d. 511 keV photons are emitted perpendicular to each other.

False: The 511 keV photons are emitted travelling in opposite directions to each other.

e. Emitted photons are detected by bismuth germanate (BGO) detector.

True: One of the most common detectors in PET imaging is BGO.

Q8.15 Positron emission tomography III

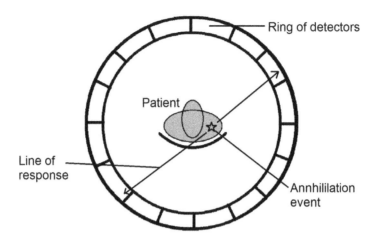

Positron decay occurs when an atomic nucleus is unstable due to an excess of protons (excess positive charge). The nucleus is stabilised by the decay of a proton to a neutron and the emission of a positron.

$$P^+ = n + e^+ + \nu + energy$$

where, p^+ is a proton, n is a neutron, e^+ is a positron, and ν is a neutrino.

In positron emission tomography (PET) imaging (true or false)

a. The most commonly used positron emitter is ^{18}F.

b. Positrons are emitted during an annihilation process.

c. Scintillation detectors are used to detect emitted positrons.

d. 511 keV photons are detected coincidentally.

e. Annihilation photons are detected in detectors perpendicular to each other.

Answers

a. The most commonly used positron emitter is ^{18}F.

True: The fluorine element is the most commonly used because of the ease with which it can be used in conjunction with a carrier molecule, however, other nuclides are positron emitters, for example, ^{11}C isotope.

b. Positrons are emitted during an annihilation process.

False: High energy photons are emitted at the annihilation process.

c. Scintillation detectors are used to detect emitted positrons.

False: Scintillation detectors are used to detect emitted high energy photons.

d. 511 keV photons are detected coincidentally.

True: Yes, although there are three types of incident events (true coincidence, random coincidence and scatter coincidence).

e. Annihilation photons are detected in detectors perpendicular to each other.

False: The detectors are formed in a ring within the gantry of the PET scanner. The detectors opposite each other collect the incident photons.

Q8.16 Isotopes

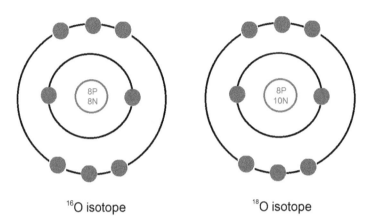

^{16}O isotope ^{18}O isotope

Isotopes are defined as variants of a chemical element which differ in neutron number. As a result of this they differ in the number of nucleons (individual particles in the nucleus). Each isotope of the same element will have a different atomic mass compared to the standard for that element (for example, oxygen has an isotope with 18 nucleons, whereas the 'standard' element has 16 nucleons). Stable isotopes do not decay, whereas unstable isotopes decay to create a new element.

Concerning isotopes of radionuclides (true or false)
   a. All isotopes of an element have the same number of protons.
   b. All isotopes of the same element have the same number of neutrons.
   c. Carbon-13 has six protons and seven neutrons.
   d. They may be unstable due to an excess of neutrons.
   e. Molybdenum-98 is made unstable by the removal of a neutron.

Answers

    a. All isotopes of an element have the same number of protons.

        True: The variation in atomic mass for isotopes of the same element is due to the different number of neutrons.

    b. All isotopes of the same element have the same number of neutrons.

        False: It is the variation in neutrons that creates new isotopes of the same element.

    c. Carbon-13 has six protons and seven neutrons.

        True: Carbon atomic number is 6 (the most common isotope has six neutrons).

    d. They may be unstable due to an excess of neutrons.

        True: Unstable nuclei generally have an excess of one or two neutrons in the nucleus.

    e. Molybdenum-98 is made unstable by the removal of a neutron.

        False: Molybdenum-98 is a stable isotope.

Q8.17 Radionuclide imaging I

Imaging using isotopes is conventionally referred to as radionuclide imaging (RNI). The technique is valuable for identifying elevated tissue function but this may arise from one or more possible alternatives. Tissue function is therefore a factor in image contrast but so is the isotope used and the carrier pharmaceutical and hence RNI is a complex technique but one which has proven utility in managing complex patient conditions.

When considering your choices in the use of isotopes (true or false)
  a. One reason for choosing technetium as an imaging isotope, is for its gamma ray energy which is close to that the optimal value for the scintillator.
  b. The isotope specific activity varies with carrier pharmaceutical.
  c. Daughter products of clinically useful radiopharmaceuticals present a major risk to the patient.
  d. Dynamic scans of the kidneys are best achieved using I131 because the organ dose is low.
  e. For isotopes that are associated with specific studies such as that of the bones, there is no need to take into account the dose to the rest of the body since there is very little systemic radiation.

Answers

a. One reason for choosing technetium as an imaging isotope, is for its gamma ray energy which is close to that the optimal value for the scintillator.

   True: Matching the photon energy to the peak in absorption results is maximising sensitivity and hence reduced dose to the patient.

b. The isotope specific activity varies with carrier pharmaceutical.

   False: The specific activity of the isotope is the activity divided by the mass.

c. Daughter products of clinically useful radiopharmaceuticals present a major risk to the patient.

   False: Appropriate isotopes and carrier pharmaceuticals are chosen to prevent risks from either the decay products, or drug byproducts.

d. Dynamic scans of the kidneys are best achieved using I131 because the organ dose is low.

   False: Iodine is not used for renal studies. Iodine will preferentially locate in the thyroid which may reduce kidney exposure but renograms are usually performed using Tc.

e. For isotopes that are associated with specific studies such as that of the bones, there is no need to take into account the dose to the rest of the body since there is very little systemic radiation.

   False: Even though localisation does result in a high dose to the organ of interest, there will be whole body effects due to scatter, circulation of the isotope in the period before localisation has occurred and irradiation of tissue adjacent to the site of interest.

Q8.18 Radionuclide imaging II

Positron emission tomography is a radionuclide imaging technique that is of great value for many investigations including staging in oncology. It utilises isotopes that are positron emitters and which generally have short half-lives that make their generation and distribution to the user more complex than those used for other RNI techniques such as single photon emission computed tomography (SPECT).

With spatial resolution (true or false)
- a. PET imaging can be corrected by the absorption data derived from a CT image.
- b. The septa used between the detectors in PET are thick because of the high energy of the gamma radiation used for imaging.
- c. Spatial resolution in PET is improved by the use of high energy positrons.
- d. Reducing the coincidence window in PET degrades the system sensitivity.
- e. PET resolution is generally better than that of SPECT.

Answers

a. PET imaging can be corrected by the absorption data derived from a CT image.

True: CT can be used to calculate the attenuation properties of the tissue within a slice and can therefore also be used to correct for absorption of the gammas generated from the positron annihilation.

b. The septa used between the detectors in PET are thick because of the high energy of the gamma radiation used for imaging.

False: PET does not require septa because the only recorded signal is that from opposite detectors recorded in incidence with each other.

c. Spatial resolution in PET is improved by the use of high energy positrons.

False: One key factor in PET resolution is how far the positron travels before annihilation. This distance increases with high energy positrons and hence degrades resolution.

d. Reducing the coincidence window in PET degrades the system sensitivity.

True: If the coincidence window is very short, even those true gammas emitted from a single annihilation event will not be recorded because if not exactly in the mid-point between detectors, they will arrive at slightly different times.

e. PET resolution is generally better than that of SPECT.

True: PET resolution is comparable to or better than SPECT.

Q8.19 Positron emission tomography IV

Spatial resolution is one consideration when assessing the performance of an imaging system. There are many factors that affect the imaging resolution and these include the design and operation of the imaging system itself, artefacts such as movement of the patient and reconstruction choices such as those selected for rapid imaging. There is a theoretical limit to the spatial resolution that an imaging system can achieve as a result of the underlying scientific principles. This theoretical limit cannot be improved upon however good the design of the imaging system.

Regarding effects on resolution (true or false)
  a. High energy positrons make the region of interest look larger than it really is.
  b. PET resolution is typically around 2 lp mm^{-1}.
  c. Contrast is more important than resolution in PET images.
  d. PET resolution can be improved by the use of post-processing.
  e. Information obtained during the CT stage can be used to correct for attenuation in PET images.

Answers

a. High energy positrons make the region of interest look larger than it really is.
   True: Because the positrons will travel further if they have high energy, the volume from which they appear to arise will also increase.

b. PET resolution is typically around 2 lp mm^{-1}.
   False: PET resolution is generally much poorer than that associated with CT and typically is around 2 lp cm^{-1}.

c. Contrast is more important than resolution in PET images.
   True: Functional imaging requires a signal to be generated from enhanced activity rather than from specific anatomical boundaries. Ideally, a high resolution would be desirable but contrast sensitive to the presence of PET isotope uptake is of prime relevance.

d. PET resolution can be improved by the use of post-processing.
   False: What can be improved is a prediction of where the activity is centred, but this takes into account numerous assumptions.

e. Information obtained during the CT stage can be used to correct for attenuation in PET images.
   True: CT can be used to develop an attenuation map of the imaged slice and can therefore also be used to calculate corrections of the gamma ray attenuation.

Q8.20 Positron emission tomography V

Hybrid imaging is conceptually straightforward in that it utilises the images from two or more modalities and combines them in a manner selected by the user. A common and well-established example is PET-CT where functional and anatomical images are combined to enable the identification of which anatomical regions have elevated function. How the two images are overlayed or fused can be user selectable and developing techniques permit the mathematical generation of a true third image rather than the more simple overlay technique.

In hybrid imaging (true or false)
- a. Hybrid imaging with MRI is not possible due to the high magnetic fields affecting the performance of the second technique.
- b. Hybrid imaging usually utilises a functional technique and an anatomical technique.
- c. Ultrasound cannot be used for hybrid imaging since it is inherently a real-time technique.
- d. Registration of images in hybrid techniques must be regularly checked to avoid image errors.
- e. In hybrid imaging the two images must be acquired simultaneously to avoid errors arising from patient motion.

Answers

   a. Hybrid imaging with MRI is not possible due to the high magnetic fields affecting the performance of the second technique.

      False: MRI can be used but the interaction of the magnetic field is a severe constraint. It limits the electronics that can be used and may also require a large separation of the individual imaging modalities.

   b. Hybrid imaging usually utilises a functional technique and an anatomical technique.

      True: But this is not an absolute requirement. Hybrid imaging is a useful technique to spatially locate elevated function but there are applications whereby the chemical map generated by MR is used with CT.

   c. Ultrasound cannot be used for hybrid imaging since it is inherently a real-time technique.

      False: Ultrasound can be used in techniques such as elastography and in fact, Duplex imaging is theoretically a hybrid technique that overlays blood flow data on top of anatomical data.

   d. Registration of images in hybrid techniques must be regularly checked to avoid image errors.

      True: Any mismatch between the two images can significantly degrade the diagnostic potential of the hybrid image. The concerns arise from errors in both position and relative magnification.

   e. In hybrid imaging the two images must be acquired simultaneously to avoid errors arising from patient motion.

      False: The images can be acquired at separated time intervals so long as registration remains reliable. True simultaneous imaging is very difficult to achieve since one technique usually lies adjacent to the other and hence one is performed first even if only by a few seconds.

IOP Publishing

Scientific Basis of the Royal College of Radiologists Fellowship (2nd Edition)

Illustrated questions and answers

Malcolm Sperrin and John Winder

Chapter 9

Functional and molecular imaging

Q9.1 Molecular imaging

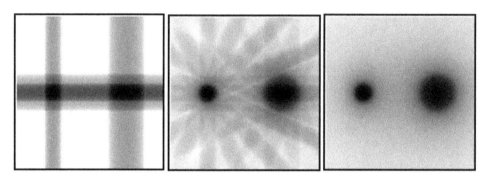

Single photon emission tomography (SPECT) is to nuclear medicine what computed tomography is to x-ray imaging. The SPECT system was in development as early as the 1970s, however, it took much longer than CT to come into clinical practice. SPECT is a technique whereby multiple cross-section images (slices) are acquired, therefore removing the effect of overlying and underlying tissue radioactivity. This leads to an increase in image contrast but also an increase in image noise. Gamma camera heads with sodium iodide crystal and photomultiplier tube detectors are rotated around the patient and gather absortion data. Images are reconstructed from this raw data.

Single photon emission computed tomography (SPECT) (true or false)
  a. Uses the same reconstruction algorithms as computed tomography.
  b. The gamma cameras may be configured with one, two or three heads.
  c. The absorption data requires correction for depth attenuation effects.
  d. The voxel size is 0.3–0.6 mm.
  e. Can produce axial, coronal and sagittal reformatted images.

Answers

a. Uses the same reconstruction algorithms as computed tomography.

   True: SPECT uses filtered back projection (as does CT), however, this method is being superseded by iterative reconstruction techniques.

b. The gamma cameras may be configured with one, two or three heads.

   True: There are single-, double- and triple-headed Gamma cameras that can perform SPECT. Multi-headed systems enable the more rapid acquisition of images or can be used for image averaging as required.

c. The absorption data requires correction for depth attenuation effects.

   True: Radioactivity from deep within the body is absorbed more strongly than radioactivity closer to the skin surface. A correction of activity with depth is routinely applied to SPECT image data to enable more accurate radionuclide concentration.

d. The voxel size is 0.3–0.6 mm.

   False: The voxel size in SPECT may be as large as 6–8 mm. A large voxel size helps reduce noise levels but also reduces spatial resolution in comparison to other imaging modalities such as CT and MRI.

e. Can produce axial, coronal and sagittal reformatted images.

   True: A volume of data may be acquired by SPECT, where slices are individually acquired and stacked together. Image reformatting in any plane is possible with the appropriate software.

Q9.2 Functional and molecular imaging I

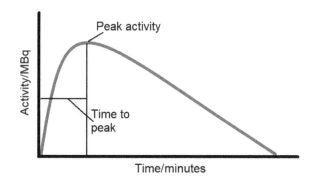

When an isotope is administered to a patient, the concentration of that isotope will increase at the site of interest in a manner that depends upon the local metabolism, excretion, carrier pharmaceutical as well as other subtle effects, including the radioactive half-life. In magnetic resonance imaging, multiple images are acquired after the injection of a contrast agent. The subjective assessment of enhancement curves may aid differential diagnosis of lesions. Semi-quantitative analysis of time intensity curves may be useful but does depend on image acquisition parameters.

In dynamic imaging studies (true or false)
  a. A time activity curve will require correction for background activity.
  b. A region of interest (ROI) is drawn over an organ to measure its radio-activity over time.
  c. Mean transit time measurements require thorough mixing of an agent with the blood before a measurement is carried out.
  d. A bolus injection of a radioactive agent will become more concentrated as it passes through the heart and lungs.
  e. CINE presentation of images is called a 'functional image'.

Answers

a. A time activity curve will require correction for background activity.

True: Background correction is required to remove activity not directly related to the organ of interest.

b. A region of interest (ROI) is drawn over an organ to measure its radioactivity over time.

True: A region of interest (ROI), is a user drawn area on an image to define the tissue or anatomy where the activity measurements should be made.

c. Mean transit time measurements require thorough mixing of an agent with the blood before a measurement is carried out.

False: A mean transit time is carried out as a bolus of contrast medium passes through the body.

d. A bolus injection of a radioactive agent will become more concentrated as it passes through the heart and lungs.

False: A bolus of radioactivity will become more mixed with blood as it passes through the heart and lungs.

e. CINE presentation of images is called a 'functional image'.

False: A CINE presentation of images creates the impression of movement or activity over time, whereas a functional image presents data of measurements across an anatomical area.

Q9.3 Optical imaging

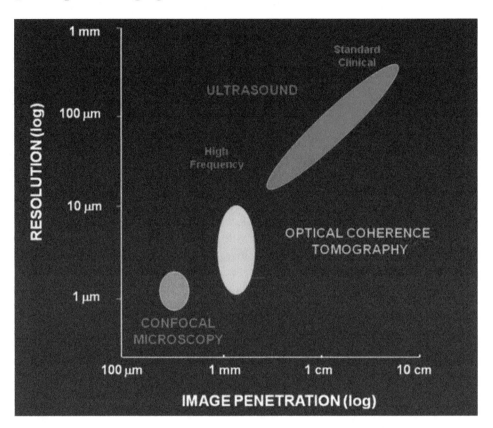

It is very common for imaging to be based on ionizing radiation as well as non-ionizing radiation such as MRI or ultrasound. In the simplest sense, this permits the investigation of internal structures without the need for intervention and thus reduces the impact and risk to the patient. It is also possible to image using optical techniques—not necessarily visible, and although there is very little scope for imaging at depth familiar to x-rays the resolution is usually very high and provides information complementary to that from the more familiar options.

With regard to imaging in the visible spectrum (true or false)
    a. The effective imaging depth of optical techniques in the visible spectrum is typically 30 mm.
    b. Fluorescence imaging presents a risk from ionizing radiation.
    c. Bioluminescence is a useful technique for identifying tissue type.
    d. Optical imaging can be associated with powers that present a risk to the patient.
    e. Optical techniques can have resolutions many times higher than mammography.

Answers

a. The effective imaging depth of optical techniques in the visible spectrum is typically 30 mm.

  False: optical wavelengths are very heavily scattered by tissue meaning that either surface imaging or penetration to a few tens of microns can be achieved.

b. Fluorescence imaging presents a risk from ionizing radiation.

  False: Fluorescence imaging is a non-ionizing technique that can theoretically lead to tissue erythema, in practice it uses such low intensity that tissue reactions are extremely unlikely.

c. Bioluminescence is a useful technique for identifying tissue type.

  False: Tissue type may be inferred but bioluminescence does not provide effective tissue discrimination since the luminescence can have a common origin even where the tissue differs.

d. Optical imaging can be associated with powers that present a risk to the patient.

  False: Powers are achievable that can disrupt tissue as is the case with surgical lasers, but the powers used for imaging are very low and will not affect the tissue in question.

e. Optical techniques can have resolutions many times higher than mammography.

  True: Optical imaging is associated with high resolution as is a common experience using microscopes. This arises from the ease with which optical wavelengths are focused and the spatial density of the detectors used.

Q9.4 Functional and molecular imaging II

(a)   (b)   (c)

(image source https://doi.org/10.1088/0034-4885/76/9/096601)

Imaging anatomy is a very familiar concept and almost as common is functional imaging. One variant of functional imaging is diffusion weighted imaging (DWI) which bases contrast on the movement of key atomic or molecular species. This introduces complexities in the interpretation of these images since no longer does the image simply display static features, but rather displays movement as vectors which vary according to location and species.

With diffusion imaging (true or false)
  a. DWI is a useful technique in studying drug efficacy.
  b. A degraded blood–brain barrier can be imaged using DWI.
  c. Molecular and functional imaging are synonymous.
  d. Functional imaging is an inherently high spatial resolution technique.
  e. Functional imaging lends itself to dynamic studies.

Answers

a. DWI is a useful technique in studying drug efficacy.

True: Where water mobility is affected by a disease and the relevant effect of drug therapy, the efficacy of the drug can be imaged using this technique.

b. A degraded blood–brain barrier can be imaged using DWI.

True: Mobility will be affected by any barrier that is degraded in terms of function. This includes the passage of water or other species across the blood–brain barrier.

c. Molecular and functional imaging are synonymous.

False: Molecular imaging is a subset of functional imaging. However, there are many variants of functional imaging.

d. Functional imaging is an inherently high spatial resolution technique.

False: In MRI functional imaging can have a relatively high resolution although not achieving that of anatomical imaging. In radionuclide imaging techniques such as PET and SPECT the resolution is measured in lp cm^{-1} as opposed to lp mm^{-1} for conventional anatomical imaging.

e. Functional imaging lends itself to dynamic studies.

True: Dynamic studies of function are very important, although the temporal resolution obtained may not be great. It is the time varying function that can be of use in addition to the static measures of function.

Q9.5 Functional and molecular imaging III

https://doi.org/10.1088/0967-3334/35/9/R167

Functional imaging is an extremely important development arising from imaging of anatomy. The contrast is based upon what the tissue is doing rather than where it is and hence is of prime diagnostic value for neuroimaging as well as oncology studies and others. Interpretation can be challenging and resolution is usually poorer than anatomical imaging but both spatial analysis and temporal analysis provide for key information often in covariance with behavioural studies.

When considering difficulties in functional imaging (true or false)
    a. Imaging function is difficult because image contrast requires a physical presence such as an atom or molecule.
    b. Magnetic resonance angiography (MRA) is a functional imaging technique.
    c. Resolutions of 2 lp mm^{-1} are typical for MR functional imaging.
    d. Blood oxygen can be used as the basis for contrast in functional studies.
    e. Cellular structures can be studied using fMRI.

Answers

a. Imaging function is difficult because image contrast requires a physical presence such as an atom or molecule.

False: Imaging function is relatively easy to image although the image characteristics of resolution, contrast, etc, differ markedly from those of anatomical imaging.

b. Magnetic resonance angiography (MRA) is a functional imaging technique.

False: MRA uses techniques to base contrast on the presence of blood and its physical boundaries but not the dynamic flow of the blood itself. Blood flow rather that imaging the blood flow itself.

c. Resolutions of 2 lp mm^{-1} are typical for MR functional imaging.

False: Functional MRI resolution is typically 2 lp cm^{-1}. The confusion arises because although the signal spatial resolution can be 2 lp mm^{-1}, the association of the function with that location is usually much poorer.

d. Blood oxygen can be used as the basis for contrast in functional studies.

True: This is a technique known as blood oxygen level dependence (BOLD), whereby the magnetic properties of the blood vary with oxygenation state and hence can be used as a basis for image contrast.

e. Cellular structures can be studied using fMRI.

False: MRI has resolutions that enable the visualisation of structures down to a few tens of mm. Cellular structures vary in size but are typically a factor of 10 or 100 smaller.

Q9.6 Biological processes for functional and molecular imaging I

https://doi.org/10.1088/0031-9155/61/15/5587

Contrast in an image will depend upon many factors, such as the normal anatomy and the presence of disease, but can routinely be enhanced using contrast agents. These agents can be as simple as air or as complex as some of the newer agents used in MRI. Some imaging techniques permit the selection of image contrast according to pulse sequence selection such as MRI. A third option utilises the intrinsic properties of the tissue such as when blood changes its magnetic properties as a result of the change in oxygenation during metabolism—a technique known as blood oxygenation level dependent (BOLD).

With regard to intrinsic contrast agents (true or false)
    a. Inflammation in MRI can only be inferred from its effect of normal anatomical shapes and boundary positions.
    b. Tumour formation can be identified utilising molecular imaging techniques.
    c. Oxygen saturation is not possible to image because its nuclear spin is zero.
    d. Tissue damage and repair are readily imaged using functional imaging.
    e. fMRI is considered to be a high contrast technique.

Answers

a. Inflammation in MRI can only be inferred from its effect of normal anatomical shapes and boundary positions.

   False: Inflammation can also be associated with enhanced blood flow and also metabolism.

b. Tumour formation can be identified utilising molecular imaging techniques.

   True: Tumours are often associated with enhanced metabolism and changes in the molecular components.

c. Oxygen saturation is not possible to image because its nuclear spin is zero.

   True: Only those species where the nuclear spin is non-zero can be imaged. The nuclear spin links the magnetisation of the atom to the external magnetic field.

d. Tissue damage and repair are readily imaged using functional imaging.

   True: It is common for fractures, age related change, etc, to show up on RNI imaging, which can be difficult to separate from other types of tissue change.

e. fMRI is considered to be a high contrast technique.

   True: Functional imaging is usually considered to be high contrast since processing of the fMRI data permits the accurate identification of signal related to function.

Q9.7 Biological processes for functional and molecular imaging II

https://doi.org/10.1088/1741-2560/11/3/035006

Being able to image drug pathways is highly desirable and conceptually is similar to intrinsic contrast agents. The underlying assumption is that the tissue will respond to the drug in a manner that changes the contrast and can be imaged using one of a variety of treatment options. This is different from extrinsic agents in that a chemical process has occurred that modifies the tissue itself.

When imaging drug pathways (true or false)
    a. Drug efficacy can be inferred from the change in contrast in MRI images.
    b. Changes in tissue following trauma are difficult to image because the basic tissue composition has not significantly changed.
    c. Infection sites are imaged by utilising the effect of elevated temperature on the tissue relaxation processes.
    d. Extrinsic contrast agents are used to image metabolism.
    e. Functional imaging presents an enhanced risk to the patient as a result of the local metabolism being perturbed.

Answers
   a. Drug efficacy can be inferred from the change in contrast in MRI images.
      True: The effect of drugs on the function of the brain or other tissue can be imaged. This may result in changes in boundaries or imaged function.
   b. Changes in tissue following trauma are difficult to image because the basic tissue composition has not significantly changed.
      False: This is the basic premise of imaging.
   c. Infection sites are imaged by utilising the effect of elevated temperature on the tissue relaxation processes.
      False: Image contrast based upon temperature elevation is possible but is rarely used, and prone to limiting artefacts. The infection can be imaged by the enhanced uptake of isotopes as a result of raised metabolism.
   d. Extrinsic contrast agents are used to image metabolism.
      True: This is the basis of radionuclide imaging.
   e. Functional imaging presents an enhanced risk to the patient as a result of the local metabolism being perturbed.
      False: The metabolism which theoretically interacts with any contrast agent administered is in reality unaffected. The risk arises from other sources such as ionizing radiation or the magnetic field in MRI.

CPSIA information can be obtained
at www.ICGtesting.com
Printed in the USA
BVHW010932120220
572107BV00008B/210

9 780750 321464